Conflicts in Health Policy

Also from Westphalia Press

westphaliapress.org

The Idea of the Digital University

Masonic Tombstones and Masonic Secrets

Treasures of London

The History of Photography

L'Enfant and the Freemasons

Baronial Bedrooms

Making Trouble for Muslims

Material History and Ritual Objects

Paddle Your Own Canoe

Opportunity and Horatio Alger

Careers in the Face of Challenge

Bookplates of the Kings

Collecting American Presidential Autographs

Freemasonry in Old Buffalo

Original Cables from the Pearl Harbor Attack

Social Satire and the Modern Novel

The Essence of Harvard

The Genius of Freemasonry

A Definitive Commentary on Bookplates

James Martineau and Rebuilding Theology

No Bird Lacks Feathers

Earthworms, Horses, and Living Things

The Man Who Killed President Garfield

Anti-Masonry and the Murder of Morgan

Understanding Art

Homeopathy

Ancient Masonic Mysteries

Collecting Old Books

Masonic Secret Signs and Passwords

The Thomas Starr King Dispute

Earl Warren's Masonic Lodge

Lariats and Lassos

Mr. Garfield of Ohio

The Wisdom of Thomas Starr King

The French Foreign Legion

War in Syria

Naturism Comes to the United States

New Sources on Women and Freemasonry

Designing, Adapting, Strategizing in Online Education

Policy Diagnosis

Meeting Minutes of Naval Lodge No. 4 F.A.A.M

Conflicts in Health Policy

Regulation, Rhetoric, Theory, and Practice

Edited by Bonnie Stabile
George Mason University

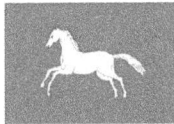

WESTPHALIA PRESS

An imprint of the Policy Studies Organization

Conflicts in Health Policy
Regulation, Rhetoric, Theory, and Practice

Westphalia Press
An imprint of Policy Studies Organization
dgutierrezs@ipsonet.org

For information:
Westphalia Press
1527 New Hampshire Ave., N.W.
Washington, D.C. 20036

ISBN-13: 978-1-935907-14-5
ISBN-10: 193590714X

Updated material and comments on this edition can be found at the Westphalia Press website: westphaliapress.org

Dedicated to Jack A. Stabile, MD

Contents

Acknowledgments

For all who share my passion for policy as colleagues, students, and friends, I am most grateful. Thanks are due to the Policy Studies Organization, especially Paul Rich and Daniel Gutierrez-Sandoval, for their support in publishing this volume, and the *World Medical & Health Policy* journal. I wish to acknowledge George Mason University's School of Public Policy, in particular the Center for the Study of International Medical Policies and Practices (CSIMPP), and credit Arnuald Nicogossian with the foresight and fortitude necessary to establish both the journal and the center. The contributions of authors and the incisive comments of reviewers and fellow editors are the lifeblood of this work, and the journal where its contents originated. With gratitude for their contributions, past, present and future, I look forward to continually working toward the diagnosis of societal ills and prescription of policy interventions, which rely upon dedicated practitioners for their application, and stalwart evaluators for their continued success.

Introduction

The study of public policy offers various tools and frameworks to enhance our understanding and improve our decision-making capacity when contending with particularly vexing problems in the public sphere, and nowhere is the need for such insight more compelling than in the area of health. Since its inception, *World Medical & Health Policy* has sought to contribute to an informed dialogue on what at times seem to be intractable policy problems dealing with health. This volume highlights contributions that make inroads in that regard, applying the language of policy scholarship to enhance understanding of health policy issues and the possibility of improved outcomes.

Clemons, McBeth, and Kusko highlight the role of policy narratives in policy development in the case of obesity, while Denis and Whitford consider presidential rhetoric and policy outcomes in the case of heroin abuse. In both instances, the study of the role of language and the power of political persuasion is elucidating, whether the language is used by the president from the bully pulpit regarding drug addiction, or in the broader public when driven by divisive symbols and emotional narratives characteristic of morality debates, in the case of obesity. In examining another form of political persuasion, Tolchin, Das Gupta, and Beck consider the importance of patronage – "the awarding of discretionary favors in government in exchange for political support" – and its role in apportioning funds to study cures or locate health care facilities for reasons of political obligation rather than public wellbeing.

The chapter on stem cells, cloning, and political liberalism serves to illustrate both the benefits and the limitations of elegant models of political philosophy, such as those admitted by Rawls in his discussion of burdens of judgment and their impact on public reason.

Where United States' domestic policy is concerned, Rudder and Fritschler's examination of the policy process surrounding the regulation of smoking and tobacco identifies six political lessons for science professionals in effectively using scientific research to inform public policy in democratic societies, recognizing that beyond scientific evidence alone, the power of persuasion—in rhetoric and narrative—is needed to effect policy change. Caulkins, Kasunic, and Lee project potential outcomes of specific proposals for marijuana legalization at the state level in 2012, and possible lessons for the nation regarding price, use, and health consequences.

In the international arena, Farinella, Saitta, and Signorino consider the implications of devolution and local government autonomy in Italy's public health system by examining the network for stroke care. Kelekar similarly examines the effects of decentralization on the structure of healthcare delivery and funding by focusing on fiscal interactions among local government units in the Philippines. These studies underscore the importance of governance structures in influencing health policy outcomes.

Finally, Campbell takes a global comparative view in examining national and regional differences in approaches to managing obesity, noting the importance of contextual values in policy interventions.

Each study highlights insights and lessons of general interest to those striving to understand and influence a broad array of health policy problems, whether through persuasion, patronage, or manipulation of the mechanisms of provision. All in some way take into account the complex element of human behavior in shaping not only human health itself, but the policies designed to manage and improve it.

Bonnie Stabile, George Mason University

Foreword

As we have argued for the past dozen years, public policy analysis is not a rational process. Rationality asserts that policy actors should first define policy problems through the careful weighing of evidence. Next, the actors build a comprehensive list of alternatives and then project the outcomes of those alternatives before choosing the optimum solution. The analyst in this model conducts research neutrally uninfluenced by his or her own subjective beliefs and values, or those of others.

While rationality remains an important element of the discipline, and thus a mixed methodological approach is needed, we have made the case that a variety of factors limit the use of the rational mode of analysis, including human intellectual and analytical limitations, the nature of political systems and organization, and political ideology and beliefs. Despite strong evidence in a variety of fields, such as cognitive psychology, which suggest that humans are not always or even predominantly rational creatures, many analysts are hesitant to accept the limitations of rationality and continue to subscribe to an entirely rational model of analysis.

Medical and health policy can easily be viewed through this lens, which views policy issues as technical problems. An analyst looking through this lens might suggest that if people are obese, we should have governmental policies to help them fight this condition. Similarly, drug abuse should be ameliorated using whatever policies have been shown to reduce such use, healthcare facilities should be funded and located based on rational studies and a rational view of the public interest, decisions on stem cells and cloning should be based solely on scientific evidence, and if cigarettes harm citizens' health then citizens will simply support cigarette regulation out of self-interest. Such views are misinformed. Medical and health policy decisions, both nationally and globally, are not formed within the context of objectivity and science but rather are determined based on beliefs, value conflict, morality, political patronage, and ethical debates. Unfortunately, many advocates, policymakers, scientists, and others still subscribe to the very rational approach to both the public policy process and public policy analysis.

We have observed that when wrestling with public policy problems and weighing proposed policy solutions and strategies, interested parties—citizens, activists, pundits, medical and scientific experts, and all too often even policy scholars and students, expect, desire, argue for, and try to utilize approaches that are purely rational, make sense scientifically, and are nonpolitical.

This is especially true when the issues: are incredibly important; are complex; are morally charged; are seemingly intractable; affect millions of people; are divisive due to conflicting values and interests; involve scarce public resources and intergovernmental relations.

These rational, scientific, nonpolitical approaches are largely doomed to failure. Science and rationality only play a limited (and sometimes limiting) role in persuading people which policy proposal makes sense. Therefore policy entrepreneurs need to learn how to:

• analyze the specific policy environment;
• craft an effective narrative;
• control the definition of the problem;
• frame the issue wisely;
• expand issue relevance and/or who is considered a stakeholder;
• venue shop.

This new health policy book, comprised of nine peer-reviewed articles that can function alone and as a cohesive whole, demonstrates why this is true, explores implications of the rational model's failure, and presents alternative models of analysis.

The chapters in this book deal with health issues such as stem cell research and cloning, obesity, stroke networks, drug addiction, marijuana legalizations, and tobacco policy. Thus, readers will be exposed to significant and timely issues in clear and concisely written chapters. More importantly, it makes clear that theory and political philosophy matter when dealing with these wicked problems. It shows that political acumen matters, because the policy arena is not free from politics, partisanship, patronage, personal political interests, bureaucratic politics and red tape, inequitable access to resources, and value-based decisions about centralization/decentralization. This is why policy experts—not just subject matter experts—need to be involved in policy advocacy efforts, policy design, policy implementation, and policy evaluation, and why this book deserves widespread readership and course-adoption.

Randy S. Clemons, Mercyhurst University
Mark K. McBeth, Idaho State University

I. Obesity Policy

The Context for Government Regulation of Obesity Around the Globe: Implications for Global Policy Action

Amy T. Campbell, JD, MBE,
Cecil C Humphreys School of Law, University of Memphis

Introduction

In our economically fraught and turbulent times, national leaders are inclined to say, "At least we're not like *them*." And yet, many of our governmental responses have similarities in form, function, and intent. Too, we see issues that transcend boundaries, issues such as obesity,[1] where we see government responses that build on what others have done, e.g., taxing unhealthy products or behaviors. It is these latter commonalities that this article addresses, namely: what does a comparative snapshot tell us about why and how governments regulate obesity, and about how context may shape or influence seemingly similar approaches.

How has obesity come to dominate so much of the international dialogue? First, there are the numbers: "OECD [Organisation for Economic Co-operation and Development] projections suggest that more than two out of three people will be overweight or obese in some OECD countries by 2020" (OECD 2012a). Costs to insurers and employers for obesity-related conditions extend well into billions, per country (Federal Ministry 2007; Finkelstein et al. 2009; 2010; Harvard School of Public Health 2012; CDC 2012c). This does not even address the less quantifiable costs for individuals and families. Numbers gain importance due to the negative health impacts of overweight and obesity on children and adults, with obesity-related conditions causing significant morbidity and mortality (CDC 2012b). So too have emotional costs been noted (Puhl and Heuer 2010).

As such costs increase, governments across the globe—even if not typically inclined to address what may be seen as individual or market factors—have responded in a myriad of ways. Approaches may focus on individuals, populations, or industry, and may lean heavier on use of "carrots" or "sticks" with financial or non-economic incentives. Taxes (explicit or implicit, e.g., "subsidy" for "good" behavior) are a frequent strategy—but may be more human-oriented (e.g., tax on individual for "choices" made) or product-oriented (e.g., tax on saturated fat or sugar content). Related to this is more or less emphasis on private actor action, and the extent of government (dis)-incentive on such action. Private or public focus, the government's role (however limited) may, in turn, concentrate its efforts at the macro (e.g., federal policy), meso (e.g., school district policy), or micro (e.g., individual fitness) level.

Some common trends have emerged in these approaches, such as the role of political pressure in adapting or rejecting certain regulatory approaches, the greater ease in "protecting children" than targeting adults, and the trumpeting of economic incentives to alter behaviors. Moreover, while evidence-based policy may be a convenient catchphrase, the reality as played out in context may be something quite different. Comparing

---

[1] It has been noted that metabolic dysfunction is the better target than obesity in and of itself (Lustig, Schmidt, and Brindis 2012); however, as obesity is the focus in much of the literature and policies, it is used herein.

approaches across settings clarifies this point—that language matters, and this language embeds within it a historical and socio-cultural context as much as seemingly objective facts.

This article offers a comparative snapshot to emphasize the important role of regional and national context in shaping government responses to obesity. It begins in Part I by setting the contextual stage for government action, focusing on a select group of individual developed nations: the United States, the United Kingdom (specifically England), France, Germany, Denmark, Australia, and Japan. Obesity numbers per country are shared, as are some comments on contextual (political, historical, and socio-cultural) factors potentially triggering and shaping government attempts to control behaviors. Next, Part II discusses recent literature on why and how law gets involved in obesity debates generally, offering select overarching frameworks as informed by public health and policy literature to guide the current discussion.

With this foundation laid, Part III explores common government responses:[2] information disclosure and use of economic incentive, with the latter broken down into taxation/subsidy on goods or industries and taxation on individuals via insurance schemes. The purposes herein are not to debate which approach is preferred and why, but rather to suggest that context impacts how given approaches are implemented, and presented to the public as necessary or helpful. Some trends and themes are identified based on this snapshot. The article concludes in Part IV with thoughts on the hope for—or value in—a global governmental response to obesity, with implications not only simply for existing efforts (e.g., United Nations (UN) and World Health Organization (WHO) work (De Schutter 2011; UN 2011; WHO 2008; 2004)), but also for what can be learned from more localized efforts (the latter the focus of this article).

It is argued that we can and should learn from each other, while also taking into account the critical role of context in tailoring regional and intra-national response.[3] Each nation (and sub-nation) has its own unique values informing its actions, values that should be acknowledged as affecting how a policy intervention is chosen, is implemented, is advocated for, is targeted, and is evaluated as "effective" vis-à-vis obesity. That is, contextual values determine "value" in policy interventions. More perspectives on determining value (quantifiable) behind given policy interventions to affect obesity can be a benefit, but only if these additional values (culturally-imbued) are understood.

Methods

Nations included within this snapshot were chosen based on the author's area of expertise and scholarship (United States), and also ones with recent news prominence in the obesity debate (United Kingdom, Denmark, and France). Another nation (Germany) was added to complement the European discussion with another governance and health system model in a nation with a different political heritage. Two additional nations were chosen (Australia and Japan) to expand the geographic diversity. One nation (Japan) was specifically featured given its unique legal approaches but low obesity rate.

---

[2] There are a myriad of areas government could seek to impact, including environmental and corporate influences on obesity; the focus, herein, however, is on information and economic incentive-related responses.
[3] For a richer understanding of how context may affect causal mechanisms/explanations in policy, see Falleti and Lynch (2009).

While not a scientific process for selection, the goal, again, was to offer a snapshot of some leading approaches across developed, OECD-member nations. By this selection, comparability is enhanced given roughly similar government traditions and/or health systems and/or economic strengths and/or "clout" in global discussion. It is recognized, however, that developing nations are also witnessing growing obesity rates, with potential divergent causes and responses. While their issues are beyond the scope of this current article's snapshot, investigation of their contexts—individually and comparatively—merits further investigation.

I. Setting the Stage: The Context for Government to Address Obesity

Obesity Data

Rising rates and costs of obesity have increasingly triggered government response; thus it is critical to have a sense of the figures. For measurement purposes herein, obesity is defined as a BMI of 30+ (kg/m^2), with overweight falling in the range of 25–29.9 BMI (CDC 2012d; WHO 2011).[4] See Tables 1 and 2 for OECD member nation obesity rates (discussed in more detail below).

---

[4] It has been argued that BMI is not an ideal marker for overweight/obesity (Rothman 2008); notwithstanding these criticisms, as this is the measure most commonly used around the globe for obesity rates, it is used herein.

Table 1
Obesity Rates Among OECD-Member and Other Nations*

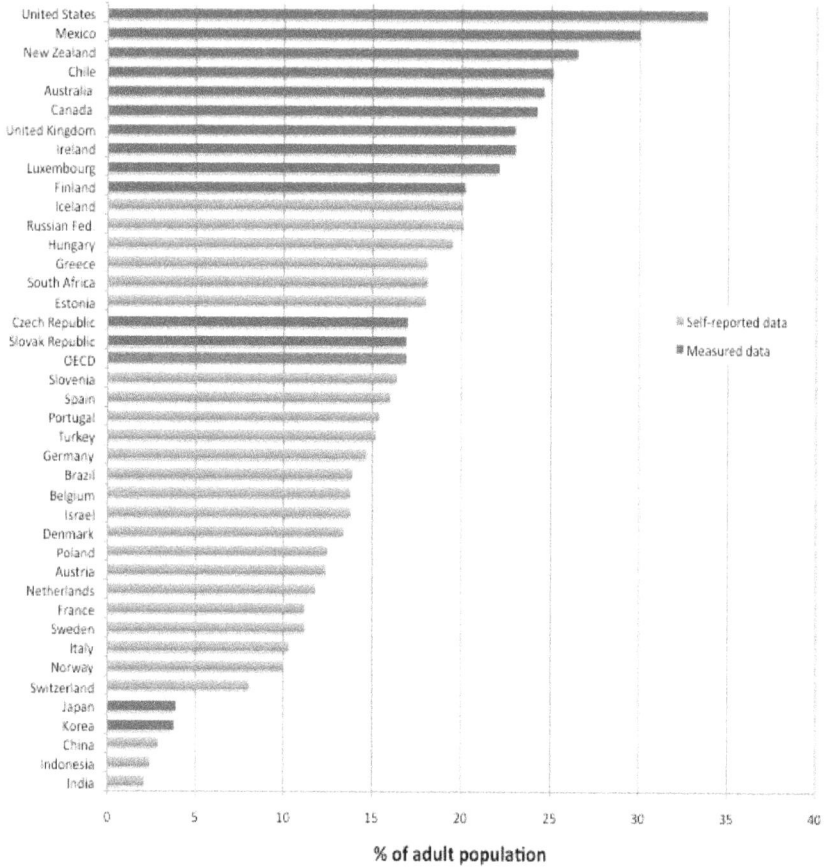

% of adult population

*Adapted with permission from OECD (2012a). Data from *OECD Health Data 2011* (OECD-member nations) and national sources (non-OECD countries).

Table 2
Obesity Rates Among Select OECD-Member Nations*

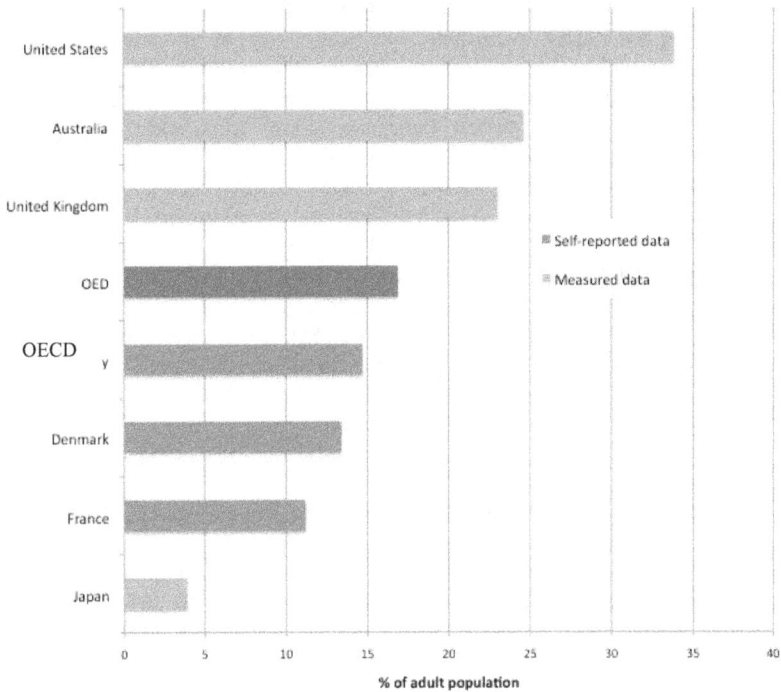

*Adapted with permission from OECD (2012a). Data from *OECD Health Data 2011* (OECD-member nations) and national sources (non-OECD countries). "Select" = covered in this article.

United States
   As of 2010, approximately 1/3 (33.8%) of U.S. adults were obese (OECD 2012a), while almost 1/5 (17%) of children (ages 2–19) were obese (CDC 2012a). The adult rates rise to 68% if overweight is added to obesity (CDC 2012f).[5] Raw numbers tell only part of the story; perhaps more critically for triggering government action are the costs associated with this prevalence. In the United States, in 2006, per capita medical spending on an obese person across all payers was 42% more than on "normal" weight peers (Finkelstein 2009). Obesity-related conditions represented an estimated 9.1% of annual U.S. medical expenditures in 2008 (*USA Today* 2009), costing employers U.S.D$73.1 billion per year (Finkelstein et al. 2010).

---

[5] The OECD has also tracked U.S. rates, indicating the United States leading position among OECD nations for its rates, with troubling trend lines (OECD 2012b). Interestingly, however, it also highlights that socio-economic disparities in the United States among those represented in obesity numbers are smaller than in other OECD nations (OECD 2012b).

Europe: United Kingdom (England), France, Germany, and Denmark

Among European nations, the United Kingdom historically has had the highest rates of obesity and overweight (OECD 2012a). In the United Kingdom, an estimated 23% of adults were obese in 2009 (OECD 2012a). The rate of obesity among the French—historically among the lowest in Europe—has been rising, to an estimated 10% of the population; factoring in overweight, this rises to 40% (OECD 2012c). As of 2009, Germany's self-reported obesity rates among adults were 14.7% (OECD 2012a). One study ranked Germany highest among European nations when adding overweight and obesity numbers (Spiegel Online International 2007). Finally, in Denmark, while self-reported obesity rates among adults increased to 13.4% in 2009 (OECD 2012a), rates are lower than those in the United States, United Kingdom, and Germany.

Other: Australia and Japan

In Australia, as of 2007–2008, 61% of adults were overweight or obese, with the greatest increase since 1995 among obese (19–24%) (Australian Bureau of Statistics 2011; Australian Government 2008a). In contrast to nations discussed thus far, Japanese obesity rates are among the lowest of OECD nations, with a rate of 3.9% among adults (OECD 2012a).

Summary

In sum, all nations (except perhaps Japan) have evidence of rising rates of obesity in the past 20+ years, trends that have often been attached to cost numbers. The OECD reports that 1–3% of total health expenditures (5–10% in the United States) may be attributed to obesity-related costs in most OECD countries (OECD 2012a). The UN, too, has recognized a concerning rise in non-communicable disease burden costs, including those related to obesity (UN 2011). These numbers, in turn, have influenced if and how national and transnational governing bodies will respond. Noteworthy, too, is the disparate representation of more vulnerable populations (e.g., low-income, racial and ethnic minorities) among obese numbers, which potentially affects the nature of governmental action (OECD 2012a). Before turning to responses, however, it is also important to situate these trends in a deeper context—that of the socio-cultural and political influences of the target nations[6]—to enhance understanding of government actions to regulate (or not) obesity, as affect whom, and with what justification.

Health Insurance System Context

Table 3 identifies select major features of the various health systems of nations making up this snapshot. For purposes herein, it is critical to note that most emphasize a more public approach to health insurance coverage, with the United States the outlier in its predominance of private (primarily employer-based) health insurance (Commonwealth Fund 2011) and in separating out coverage by age and income level (Schoen et al. 2010, 2324). Publicly financed healthcare in the United States includes Medicare (primarily old age), Medicaid (primarily low income), Children's Health Insurance, and TriCare (veteran's health) programs, illustrating the lack of unity even within the publicly

---

[6] What follows is not intended to be a deep analysis of cultural and political trends in the nations; rather, the goal is to highlight the importance of a richer understanding of such context to understand the favored approaches among governments—as developed, as implemented, and as reported upon and experienced by individual, population, and corporate stakeholders. Readers interested in more information about the various political/governmental structures are referred to the great number of policy journals.

financed health system. In fact, the United States has been noted for its fragmentation and significant numbers of un- and underinsured (Schoen et al. 2010). Among European nations, healthcare coverage is typically provided through national health insurance (social citizenship based-entitlement—England, Denmark) or statutory health insurance (France, Germany). Japan, too, implements a statutory health insurance scheme, while Australia offers universal public insurance via its Medicare program.

Table 3
Select Features of Health Insurance Systems*

Health System	United States	England	France	Germany	Denmark	Australia	Japan
Government Insurance Role[a]	OTH	NHS	SHI	SHI	NHS	UPI	SHI
Private Insurance Role[b]	5	1	2	3/4	3	3	3/4
Nature of Public Financing[c]	PT, FT, ST, Pr	GTR	EEIT, EEPT, GTR	EEPT, GTR	EIT	GTR, EIT	GTR, Pr
Nature of Provider Payment[d]	FFS, Some C	C/P4P mix; S (public)	FFS	FFS	FFS/C	FFS	FFS
Primary Care Role[e]	G (some)	G, R	G (national incentives)	G (some)	G, R	G	
Seek to Enhance Competition Among Insurers	Y			Y			

*Adapted with permission from Tables 1 and 4 and country profiles of Commonwealth Fund 2011; see also Schoen et al. 2010. Descriptions approximate.

[a]SHI: Statutory Health Insurance; NHS: National Health Service; UPI: Universal public insurance program; OTH: Other.
[b](author-determined continuum): 5: At least ½ population access PHI coverage; 1: Low % accesses PHI coverage for certain amenities; 2: Use PHI to cover out-of-pocket expenses (e.g., cost-sharing); 3: Use PHI to cover out-of-pocket expenses and get additional services; and certain % opt out for full PHI; 3/4: High % access PHI for extra benefits and cover out-of-pocket expenses.[c]PT: Payroll tax; FT: Federal tax; ST: State tax; Pr: Premium; GTR: General tax revenue; EEIT: Employer/employee earmarked income tax; EEPT: Employer/employee earmarked payroll tax; EIT: Earmarked income tax.
[d]FFS: Fee-for-service; C: Capitation; P4P: Pay for performance; S: Salaried.
[e]G: Gatekeeping function; R: Registration with gatekeeper required.

One can see two key trends: the extent to which equity—at least for citizens—drives concerns for coverage, and the extent to which the mechanism to achieve universal coverage is via government control (restricting choice of insurer) or a more corporatist or otherwise options-driven approach (government helps fund system but does not dictate insurer choice). All systems utilize some sort of tax revenue to fund the system, but differ in sources upon which funds are drawn, with some favoring a more employer/employee-based taxation scheme. Most publicly funded systems, too, allow for access to private health insurance that helps cover certain out-of-pocket costs or opens up access to certain amenities (e.g., private hospital rooms), with the United Kingdom the leading nation at keeping down out-of-pocket costs (Schoen et al. 2010).

The purpose of this comparison is not to argue that any single healthcare system is "best" at addressing obesity; likely, arguments could be made on many sides. Moreover, as the ensuing discussion suggests, it is likely beyond the ability of any single health system, per se, to address obesity (i.e., not simply a "health system" issue), although some systems may have advantages for certain approaches based on their set-up, funding, and universality, etc. Yet, rather than wade into that debate, the goal is to set the health system context for government response to obesity as but one feature of a complex dynamic informing and influencing policy action.

Socio-cultural/Political Context

Key non-health contexts for policy responses to obesity begin with the most elemental: basic demographic data (Table 4). In turn, these raw numbers reside in political contexts shaped by culture and history. Table 5 provides a brief summary of key government structure factors. What critical defining features emerge? All nations are liberal democracies with executive, legislative, and judiciary functions, but with varying degrees of separation in powers. Some, like the United States and France, have stronger executives. Others, like Germany and the United Kingdom, are parliamentary systems with executives accountable to legislatures from which they emerge (versus popularly elected as in the United States and France) (Shugart 1993). Some, like the United States, Germany, and Australia, feature federalist systems with power divided between federal and state levels, impacting what level of government is accountable, to whom, and with what limits on its reach and authority. Japan is unique among democracies herein for its newer government formation, single party (factionalized) dominance for much of that time, and reliance on civil bureaucracy for governing (Masaru 1997).

Table 4
Country Demographics

Demographics[1]	U.S.	U.K.	France	Germany	Denmark	Australia	Japan
Population	313,142,419	63,047,162	65,630,692	81,305,586	5,543,453	22,015,576	127,368,088
Pop <18	24%[2]	21%[3]	22%[4]	16%[5]	22%[6]	23%[7]	16%[8]
Pop 18>65	62.9%[27]	62%[3,10]	62%[4,11]	63%[5,12]	62%[6,13]	63%[7,14]	61%[8,15]
Pop >65	13%[9]	17%[10]	16%[11]	21%[12]	16%[13]	14%[14]	23%[15]
Race[1]: White	72.4%[24]	92.1% (83.6% English; 8.6% Scottish; 4.9% Welsh; 2.9% Irish)	Ethnicity 92% French 4% Arab/N. African 2% German 1% Breton 1% Catalon	Ethnicity 91.5% German 2.4% Turkish 6.1% (Greek, Italian, Polish, Russian, Serb-Croatian)	Ethnicity 97% Danish 2%: Other Scan Other: 1% Faroset/Inuit	92%	
Black	12.6%[24]	2%					
Asian	4.8%[24]	3.1% (1.8% Indian; 1.3% Pakistani)				7%	99%
Other	6.5%[24]	2.8%					
Ethnicity	Hispanic: 16.3%[24]					0.43%[25]	
Gender: Females	50.8%	50.6%	51.5%	50.8%	50.8%	50.5%	51.6%
Males	49.2%	49.4%	48.5%	49.2%	49.2%	49.5%	48.4%
Religion[26]: Christian	78.5%	71.6%	67%	62%	82% (80.7% ELC)	64%	Many Japanese report being both Shinto and Buddhist so % of reporting: 84.7% Shinto, 69% Buddhist; 1.8% Christian; 7% Other
Jewish	1.7%	<1%	<1%*	<1%	<1%	.4%	
Buddhist	n/a	<1%	1%	<1%	<1%	2.1%	
Muslim	0.6%	3%	6–10%*	4%	3.6%	1.7%	
Not Affiliated	12.1%	23.1%	4%	33%	13%	20%	
Political Parties	Democrats 31%[16]	Labor 29%[17]					
	Republicans 29%	Conservative 36%					
	Independent 38%	Liberal Democrat 23%					
GDP Per Capita	$48,100	$35,900	$35,000	$37,900	$40,200	$40,800	$34,300
Language	English 80%[18]	English 95%[19]	French 93%[20]	German 90%[21]	Dutch 97%[22]	English 79%	Japanese 99%[23]
	Spanish 13%	Celtic >5%				Chinese 3%	
						Italian 2%	

*France has largest European Jewish and Muslim communities. Government does record ethnic statistics.

Sources:

1: All data, unless specified otherwise infra: Central Intelligence Agency 2012.
2: U.S. Census Bureau 2012.
3: Unicef 2012a.
4: Unicef 2012b.
5: Unicef 2012c.
6: Unicef 2012d.
7: Unicef 2012e.
8: Unicef 2012f.
9: U.S. Census Bureau 2012.
10: U.K. National Statistics 2012.
11: Ministére des Affaires Ètrangéres et Européennes 2008.
12: index mundi 2012.
13: European Commission/Eurostat 2011.
14: Australian Bureau of Statistics 2010.
15: Ministry of Internal Affairs and Communication 2008.
16: Gallup Politics 2011.
17: Darlington 2012.
18: U.S. Census Bureau 2010.
19: BBC 2012.
20: European Commission 2006.
21: European Commission 2006.
22: European Commission 2006.
23: School Directory 2012.
24: U.S. Census Bureau 2011a.
25: Australian Bureau of Statistics 2007.
26: U.S. Department of State 2011b.
27: U.S. Census Bureau 2011b

Table 5
Governance/Political Systems*

Political System:	United States	England	France	Germany	Denmark	Australia	Japan
Governance Structure	Federal Republic (federal/50 states); Republic Constitution Presidential	Constitutional Monarchy; Parliamentary (Westminster-style)	Republic Semi-Presidential	Federal Republic (16 federal states) Parliamentary	Constitutional monarchy Parliamentary	Constitutional Monarchy; Parliamentary; Federalist (Commonwealth and 6 States); written Constitution	Constitutional Monarchy; Parliamentary
Executive (sometimes referred to as the "government")	President—popularly elected (one round)	Monarch (head of state) -and- Prime Minister (head of government; PM drawn from majority party/coalition that wins Parliamentary election -and- Cabinet (leading decision-making body, drawn from MP and Lords (highest ranking members), selected by PM)	President, Popularly elected (two rounds; single winner) -and- Prime Minister (appt'd by President)	Federal Chancellor (*Bundeskanzler*), elected by *Bundestag*; usually part of same party holding most seats in parliament with coalition support (proportional rep) -and- President—elected by Federal Assembly; ceremonial role	Monarch -and- Prime Minister (coalition-led role)	Monarch (Queen of England; head of state), represented by Governor-General in Australia (selected by PM) -and- Prime Minister (elected through government; member of Parliament) -and- Federal Executive Council (ministerial advice to Governor-General) -and- Cabinet (PM and Ministers of State; selected by PM; majority drawn from Parliament; accountable to Parliament)	Emperor (head of state; largely ceremonial role post-WWII) -and- Prime Minister (head of government; member of Parliament and designated by it) -and- Cabinet (PM and Ministers of State; selected by PM; majority drawn from Parliament; accountable to Parliament)

Political System:	United States	England	France	Germany	Denmark	Australia	Japan
Judiciary	Independent; interpret (not make) law	Independent; interpret (not make) law	Minister of Justice; independent branch; also has powerful Constitutional Court (const'l rights/human rights violations)	Independent	Independent	Independent—High Court of Australia—interprets Constitution	Independent; Supreme Court (final authority); no jury system
Legal Tradition	Common law	Common law	Civil/codified Roman Law (*Code Civil*)	Civil	Civil	Common law	Civil (also draws from customary law, common law)
Main Political Parties	Left to Right: Democratic/Republican	Left to Right: Liberal Democrat (Clegg)/Labour/Conservative (Cameron)	Left to Right: Parti socialiste (PS)/Mouvement democrate/Union pour un mouvement populaire (UMP) (Sarkozy)	From Left to Right: Left Party/Green Party/Social Democratic Party (SDP)/Free Democratic Party (FDP)/ Christian Democratic Union (CDU), and its sister party, Christian Social Union (CSU) (Merkel)	Left to Right: Red-Green Alliance Greens/Australian Labor Party (centre-left, social democratic party, Democrats (Thorning-Schmidt)/Conservative People's Party (centre-right)/National Party (rural interests) *Note: Compulsory voting by all citizens over age of 18 in federal and state elections	Left to Right: Social Democratic Party (SDP, formerly the Socialist Party)/Democratic Party of Japan (DPJ, centre left) (Noda)/New Komeito (NKP)/Liberal Democratic Party (LDP)	Left to Right: People's Party/Socialist People's Party/Social Liberals/Social Liberals/People's populist People's Party

*Note: This author-developed table provides a broad overview and the author's best approximation of power structures and party standing.

Any errors are the author's own.

Sources:

General: Neto and Samuels 2010.

United States: Congressional Research Service 2001.

United Kingdom: Direct.gov 2012a; Direct.gov 2012b; www.parliament.uk 2012a; www.parliament.uk 2012b.

France: About-france.com 2012; Ministère des Affaires Etrangéres 2008; The Economist 2008.

Germany: Germany.co.za 2012; Australian Government 2012a.

Denmark: Denmark.dk 2012; Australian Government 2012b.

Australia: Australian Government 2012c; Parliament of Australia 2011.

Japan: U.S. Department of State 2011a; Administrative Management Bureau 2007; Web Japan 2012; Washington Post 1998.

Political System:	United States	England	France	Germany	Denmark	Australia	Japan
Legislature	Congress (bicameral): House of Representatives (lower); Senate (upper)—both popularly elected	Parliament (bicameral): House of Commons (lower house; popularly elected; party with largest # forms government; members of = MPs; controls decisions on financial bills); House of Lords (appointed)	Parliament (bicameral): *Assemblée nationale* (lower/primary)—popularly elected; *Sénat*—indirectly elected	Bicameral: *Bundestag* (lower house Parliament)—popularly elected & proportional representation; *Bundesrat* (upper house, Federal Council)—represents 16 state governments/only approves legislation affecting state responsibilities	Parliament (unicameral, *Folketing*)—popularly elected proportional representation	Parliament (bicameral)—Senate (upper house, popularly elected from states (equal rep) and territories, often controlled by minority party; thus check on House/PM); House of Representatives (lower house, popularly elected; majority party/coalition forms Government), plus Queen (rep'd by Governor-General)	Parliament (bicameral, *Diet*); House of Representatives (lower; popularly elected; can be dissolved by PM or Cabinet); House of Councillors (upper; popularly elected; cannot be dissolved)
Government power center	President & Legislature. Accountable to Constitution (supreme law of land (*and* states—federalism)	Parliament (it forms government, is check on Cabinet; can dismiss government via "no confidence" vote)	President	Parliament (*and* states—federalism)	Parliament	Cabinet—composed of senior Ministers drawn from Parliament, (decides on major policy proposals), with Prime Minister (who selects Cabinet members)	Parliament (*Diet*); in reality, civil servants wield much control (due in part to turbulence in PM leadership and long-term LDP dominance with intra-party factional debate)
Policy Made by	President (with agencies; regulatory; can veto legislation) and Legislature (make laws; can override Pres. veto)	Cabinet	President, with Council of Ministers	Cabinet (Chancellor and Federal Ministers)	PM with Cabinet (Ministers)	Cabinet	PM (over Cabinet)

Critically, for purposes herein, the United States puts great emphasis on individual rights and liberty interests, with related distrust of government attempts to control what are seen as individual behaviors or are seen as better addressed by market action (a more laissez-faire approach). Too, the importance of states in setting health policy impacts how obesity is addressed. Beyond the United States, there has historically been less emphasis on individual rights and more on communal responsibilities, more support for universal healthcare, and more inclination toward social welfarist traditions (Cousins 2005)—all critical to understand perspectives on how best to address obesity. And yet, each nation (and regions within nations) has strong traditions in its own right that at times bring about disparate approaches to healthcare. Moreover, economic challenges and "Euroscepticism" (Lubbers and Scheepers 2010; Sorenson 2008; Boomgaarden et al. 2011) render more visible tensions in approaches and philosophies, primarily between the United Kingdom, France, and Germany.

In sum, while similarities exist among OECD nations, strong national and inter-regional identities remain strong, and should be recognized and studied to better understand government action vis-à-vis obesity. One could imagine, for example, how a welfarist tradition, communitarian impulse, and universal healthcare system leveraged in part through collective taxes, might create a fertile environment for collective taxation approaches. Alternatively, a nation that is more skeptical of government intrusion in what it may see as private decisions, might be much more hesitant to allow government to impose population-level taxes for what could be viewed as the behavioral choices of individuals.

II. Regulating through Law

> "… the law can be used to create conditions that allow people to lead healthier lives and … the government has both the power and the duty to regulate private behavior in order to promote public health."
> (Mello, Studdert, and Brennan 2006, 2601 (references omitted))

Even if we recognize an obesity problem within and transcending national boundaries, how exactly does it get on a government agenda, and how in turn does this influence the framework for government response? This section addresses government's role as descriptively experienced (versus as normatively or legally defined (Gostin 2000; Swinburn 2008)). That is, the focus is on what this government role looks like (the "what is"), as contextually developed, which in turn influences how the "problem" of obesity is cast.

The How

> "Genes and culture load the gun, but the economic environment pulls the trigger." (Swinburn 2008, 2)

Getting on the Agenda

Obesity numbers—lives impacted and associated costs to individuals, societies, and governments—inform governmental action. Simple numbers may indicate a "rational" economic response to attack obesity. In reality, however, rational action driven by cost effectiveness research is much more complicated (what costs count? who decides what is effective?); too, economics is not the only driver. Other ways to become a priority in republican democracies is by earning a majority of the votes (e.g., majority of voters behind doing something about an issue), or by interest group politics (e.g., lobbying) (Goddard et al. 2006, 82-85). Also important are bureaucratic (e.g., agency, Cabinet) decision makers who may seek to concentrate and maintain their power centers (e.g., keep obesity as a health insurance or public health or agriculture policy matter). (Goddard et al. 2006, 85-86; Considine 2002). Alternatively, one may adopt a laissez-faire explanation of government action, i.e., a limited government role is still a "choice" of (in) action.

Regulating through Law: a Pathway

Once on the agenda and a priority for some sort of government response, there are many avenues by which the government can thusly act. Regarding obesity, the dilemma has often been whether it is a health issue (individual or public) or something else. Martin (2008, 4-5) sets out a helpful framework, defining the paths as following a medical, economic, social, public health, or personal problem approach.[7] Table 6 illustrates what obesity as a policy problem might look like if following the different paths.

Table 6
Obesity Path Framing*

OBESITY as	Who to Address	How to Address
Medical problem	The medical system	Treat related illnesses; encourage weight loss
Economic problem	Taxing authorities, employers, and insurers	Taxes (subsidies) on products or individuals; hiring practices; different insurance plans and wellness incentive bonuses
Social problem	Society with government backing	Create stigma around fast food eating and enhance availability of community farmers' markets
Public health problem	Public and government	Healthy behavior campaigns; enhanced access to healthy foods (and less to "fast" foods)
Personal problem	Individual	Develop individual weight loss program; pay surcharge if over certain BMI
Industry problem	Industry with government	Limit access to certain products in certain locations (e.g., schools) or for certain populations (e.g., children via advertising)
Environmental problem	Government with industry support	Create environments conducive to more walking, biking

*Based on criteria in and adapted from Martin (2008, 4-5). Modified to add industry and environmental levels.

---

[7] Not explicitly highlighted but also important are industry/market or environmental mechanisms of action as well. See, e.g., Swinburn (2008); Sacks, Swinburn, and Lawrence (2008).

Generally, movement seems to flow from one path to another as "costs" mount, or images change. With obesity, economic paths have been featured, as have public health options. For the latter, inasmuch as government has the ability to track populations (surveillance), and is able to think at a population level about how to prevent disease and promote healthy behaviors, it is natural that public health issues—which many believe a rise in obesity rates to be—would be addressed via government (legal) means (Gostin 2008; Parmet 2008; Pomeranz and Gostin 2009). This, however, creates tension within nations with a liberal state tradition of an ethic of personal responsibility and individual choice (Magnusson 2008a), hence the impact of contextual drivers and political trade winds on which approach is favored, and why. From this we see an attempt to join the public and private in a shared responsibility (Federal Ministry 2007). Finally, we may see a focus on the individual: obesity is a personal problem to address via behavioral change (incentivized by a "nudge" (Thaler and Sunstein 2008) or something more).

Critically, while a path metaphor or table depiction may make the approach seem rational and linear (or cyclical), this is a dynamic process with varying entry and exit points and evolution and adaptation in the light of emerging research, obesity data points, and the myriad of socio-cultural, economic, and political factors (a focus herein). This complexity suggests that a more systematic approach is necessary (Sacks, Swinburn, and Lawrence 2008). With this in mind, perhaps a more apt metaphor would invoke prisms—which may be overlapping and with more or less transparency—through which to view government action.

Regulating through Law: Approaches

Once government gets involved (regardless of path or prism), legal mechanisms are available to shape desired stakeholder responses to obesity. Hodge, Garcia, and Shah (2008) describe legal approaches generally as including: incentives to encourage healthy behavior or financial disincentives to discourage unhealthy[8] behavior (e.g., BMI insurance surcharges); restrictions or requirements placed on food industry (e.g., healthier options in school lunches); litigation; restrictions on access to certain foods (e.g., in schools, via use of food subsidies); regulations on information flow to consumer (e.g., menu labeling); regulations on advertising or marketing (e.g., what may be shown during children's programming hours); and insurance coverage mandates (e.g., covering obesity-related treatments).[9]

Specifics on some follow; for now, it is critical that there is a toolbox available from which to pick and choose various legal approaches to develop a comprehensive response to a complex problem (OECD 2012a, 3), approaches that are, in turn, influenced by the context in which a government acts and which shapes the philosophy by which it acts (as described above). Needed now is more evidence of effectiveness of legal interventions, with a broader and deeper appreciation of what is considered to be effective and by whom. And yet, governments are acting, despite (regardless of?) full information on which to act, actions to which this article now turns.

III. A Comparative Snapshot of Common Government Mechanisms

---

[8] Critically, the law may perceive "healthy" or "unhealthy" as objective terms describing behavior; however, this risks discounting the values and emotions embedded in such terms as experienced, self-defined, or impacted. For more on emotions and health policies like these, see Campbell (2012).

[9] See also Orszag (2008), 10-12.

As Part II illustrates, governments have at their disposal a variety of prisms through which to view the "problem" of obesity and related legal tools to effectuate goals for government intervention. These general guideposts help determine if/how the focus is on the individual, the population (or subset thereof), or industry. For the first two, in turn, it also informs characteristics used to define target populations (e.g., age, BMI level) and behavior change mechanisms. What follows are some prominent approaches across nations, starting from the (seemingly) less contentious (information) to the more so (taxation).

Information

One approach to altering behaviors is to create more informed consumers by altering the flow and scope of information. Information-related regulations include labeling requirements (promote informed consumer) and advertising restrictions (restrict information flow to certain populations at certain times). In general, there has been greater endorsement of approaches that target youth or that enhance information, versus those that restrict "speech" among industry actors.

Labeling
There have been efforts to alter what is posted on food products, and in eating establishments, with a goal to better educate consumers about their food choices. One approach accords with "truth in labeling"—labeling changes on various food items to encourage understanding of contents, or greater accuracy in stated claims (e.g., what "whole" means). If viewed along a spectrum of government "intrusion" on private actors, labeling requirements such as these might fall at the less controversial end of the continuum.

Moving along the continuum to the more controversial, potentially, are requirements for calorie counts on menu boards of chain restaurants or adjacent to foods sold in vending machines or retail stores. In the United States, the push began at a local level, e.g., New York City, which required posting of menu calorie labels by certain restaurants, effective in 2008 (Nestle 2010). While data to support the law's effectiveness in altering ultimate food purchase behaviors is mixed (Elbel et al. 2009; Dumanovsky et al. 2011), federal health reform legislation, the Patient Protection and Affordable Care Act ("ACA"), built on these efforts, making these postings a federal requirement (ACA 2010 § 4205; see also Nestle 2010). One could argue that this is an overreach; for industry, however, it could also arguably serve to unify expectations versus having to deal with a patchwork of local or state-by-state requirements, in nations with less "national government" presence/oversight. But if industry perceives itself as falling on the wrong side of the "healthy" debate, affecting (potentially) market share, unsurprisingly lobbying often ensues (Martin 2008, 7; Swinburn 2008, 5).

Advertising Restrictions
Given the strong First Amendment and freedom of speech protection in the United States, it is perhaps unsurprising that restrictions on industry advertising have been less successful—although we have seen limits on some advertising, e.g., smoking (Gostin, Arno, and Brandt 1997). Internationally, however, there is greater support for limiting marketing of products to children, who are seen as especially vulnerable to advertising pitches. The International Association for the Study of Obesity (IASO) led efforts to

develop international guidelines and recommendations around marketing to children (IASO 2012). An international meeting of the International Obesity Task Force in 2006 led to the Sydney Principles ("Principles"), which promoted marketing restrictions on energy-dense, low nutrient foods and beverages (IASO 2006). In citing the industry's inability to adequately self-regulate, the Principles endorsed a statutory, cross-border response. Too, urged were responses that reflected the myriad of ways children receive information and interact with media.

Parallel to these efforts, the United Kingdom has been particularly active in its approach to advertising regulation through its Office of Communication ("Ofcom"). It has implemented a phased-in approach to marketing restrictions of high fat, salt, or sugary foods aired during children's programming, with regulations, as of 2009, covering all children's programming and channels (Ofcom 2007). Australia, too, has regulations limiting advertising in children's programming (Handsley 2009).

BMI Reporting
Labeling and advertising primarily relate to food content and food industry action (or limits on action). Within the United States, however, there have also been efforts to inform parents and public health authorities of BMI numbers among children for tracking and informing purposes. In 2003, Arkansas became the first state to require BMI[10] reporting (on school report cards) (Arkansas Act 1220 2003; Ryan et al. 2006). Research has shown this to increase awareness—and critically, not to increase disordered eating behaviors; however, more dramatic effects are less clear (Boozman College of Public Health 2009). Another study, however, suggests that the harms from BMI reporting may exceed potential benefits (Evans and Sonneville 2009). Despite limited evidence of behavior change (versus information enhancement), at least 20 states now include BMI surveillance through schools, although more often through health certificates or exams versus on report cards (see, e.g., Conis 2010).[11]

Health Impact Assessments
Information might not only be directed at individuals; it could also enhance policymakers' actions. Health Impact Assessments (HIAs) are growing "means of accessing the health impacts of policies, plans and projects in diverse economic sectors using quantitative, qualitative and participatory techniques" (World Health Organization 2012). Applied in the context of obesity, say, an HIA could help identify if and how a policy fosters or impedes an obesogenic environment. Applied more specifically to obesity, Swinburn (2008) suggests development of an Obesity Impact Assessment for laws to encourage systematic and thoughtful attention to how a given law, even if not specifically about weight, might impact such, e.g., enhance or limit ability for walking in a given community. Joining HIAs with additional framing tools, thus, could be a means to tackle obesity at a broader level (i.e., to address government and corporate

---

[10] It has been recognized that BMI has its limitations as a marker of obesity, with other measures offered as more accurately determining obesity, e.g., testing of body fat percentage (see, e.g., Shah and Braverman 2012). However, as of this writing, BMI alone seems to have been selected by states as a convenient single measure (perhaps given the debate over other appropriate measures, and the costs that might be associated with multiple measures).

[11] While this approach seems more United States-specific, concerns about child obesity rates is a worldwide phenomenon. For example, in 2010 the German teachers' association (DL) called for regular weigh-ins of children in schools, with potential reports to child welfare authorities (The Local 2010).

responsibility in supporting and sustaining unhealthy environments) (Swinburn, Egger, and Raza 1999).

Perhaps because of limited data showing behavior change from information, many governments are going further. In times of economic distress, it should not be surprising that financial incentives would enter the debate, whether as direct government response or indirect consumer experience, and whether as autonomy promoting or justice impacting. It is to these economic incentives—couched as "taxes" or "subsidies"—to which this part now turns.

Economic Incentives: The Power to Tax, The Desire to Subsidize

> "[T]he dominant environmental drivers of obesity are economic and ... the dominant solutions will need to be policy-based." (Swinburn 2008, 2)

The costs of obesity—to human lives, to individual and family budgets, to employers, to insurers, and to governments across the globe—fuel many discussions about what, if anything, the government can or should do to rein in these costs. In the United States, the debate often looks to the impact of economics on individual liberty, especially if the costs shift to "us." Alternatively, when the costs shift to the "other," it becomes more about obligations of individual responsibility and allowing individual choice but tying costs to certain choices. Internationally, too, we see discussions of individual responsibility, but add to this a sense of solidarity, a socio-cultural phenomenon that can be seen as an outgrowth of welfare system traditions (Cousins 2005). Another perspective might use a "responsive communitarian" approach (Etzioni 2010a; Etzioni 2010b). Thus, while all nations may be driven by economic concerns, context may influence political response. Governing bodies may look more to the individual or population, or specific food or general industry, as economic target, and incorporate a tax or subsidy to encourage (or discourage) certain action.

Food/Beverage Taxes

One approach is to tax certain products, e.g., high sugar content foods or beverages, often through an excise or sales tax. An excise tax is imposed on the producer (e.g., food corporation), which tax such producer typically passes on to consumers (more or less visibly) in the form of higher prices for tax-impacted goods. A sales tax, on the other hand, is a tax placed on the consumer at the time of purchase (State of Hawaii 2000). There may be strengths and weaknesses of both in terms of ability to alter purchasing behaviors, but both entail likely higher consumer prices. This highlights a leading concern of taxation approaches: the disparate impact such may have on lower-income households and individuals (Magnusson 2008c; Brownell et al. 2009, 1603; Fletcher Frisvold, and Tefft 2010; Caraher and Cowburn 2005). Notwithstanding equity considerations, taxes on goods are prominently featured across nations.

In the United States, this has typically involved attempts to impose a sugary beverage ("soda") tax. Leading researchers have written in support of these taxes (Brownell et al. 2009; Lustig, Schmidt, and Brindis 2012). Data to support these claims specific to food/beverage products is mixed, however, (Koplan, Leverman, and Kraak

2005; Goodman and Anise 2006), although this could also be due to the difficulty in implementing such taxes broadly and long-term, limiting data collection. Others suggest that effectiveness depends on the type of tax and populations targeted (Smith, Lin, and Lee 2010; Caraher and Cowburn 2005; Allais, Bertail, and Nichèle 2010), and that additional evidence is needed (Goodman and Anise 2006; Powell and Chaloupka 2009). States like New York (Berger 2010) and cities like Philadelphia (*USA Today* 2011) have tried to impose soda taxes for economic and health reasons; efforts that have been stymied by powerful industry lobbying (Caraher and Cowburn 2005, 1247-1248; Brownell et al. 2009, 1603), by individuals who believe taxes punish their own choices (Sullum 2004), and by anti-tax sentiment (Hartocollis 2010).

Beyond the United States, other countries have had more success in imposing taxes, although the data remains mixed on how successful such will be on altering demand and changing behaviors (Goodman and Anise 2006; Allais, Bertail, and Nichèle 2010). In December 2011, the French Constitutional Court approved a higher tax on soda beverages (exempting their "diet" versions), in part to combat changing diets that are "turning the traditionally skinny French into a nation of fatties" (Watson L 2011). Money raised through the tax will help lower farm worker social security payments, a notable population to benefit. France also recently raised its VAT tax rate from 5.5% to 7% on certain "takeaway" foods, e.g., pizza and burgers (Buffery 2011), although indicating a more economic (versus health)-driven motivation.

In October 2011, Denmark took center stage in the taxation approach debate when it introduced the first reported food "fat tax" in the world (Katrandjian 2011; Kaplan 2011; BBC News 2011). Targeting a specific food content, Denmark imposed a surcharge on food made up of more than 2.3% saturated fat, stating among its reasons for doing so the need to fight obesity and heart disease, and increase life expectancy (Kaplan 2011; OECD 2012a, 4). Of note, Denmark has not been singled out among OECD nations as having a particularly obese population; yet, this is not a novel approach for Denmark: In 2004, it banned foods having more than 2% trans fat, and in 2010, it raised taxes 25% on sugary foods like ice cream (Katrandjian 2011). Since Denmark's action, David Cameron has indicated support for a potential "fat tax" in the United Kingdom as well, to target falling life expectancy and address soaring healthcare costs; notably, the United States was cited as a nation not to emulate (The Telegraph 2011).[12]

Company/Industry Subsidies (Taxes)[13]

Moving beyond select foods or beverages, certain industries or corporations have been targeted, via economic (dis)-incentive. First, industry actors may view the preceding discussion as an industry tax by taxing certain of their critical products (e.g., soda). Alternatively, however, some (e.g., farmers) may be positively affected by subsidies.

---

[12] As Cameron said, "But frankly, do we have a problem with the growing level of obesity? Yes. ...Do we have a kind of warning in terms of, look at America how bad things have got there, about what happens if we don't do anything? Yes, that should be a wake-up call" (*The Telegraph* 2011).
[13] A great deal more could be written about corporate actors' role in the "obesity epidemic," and how behaviors of corporate entities and food distributors (and their lobbyists) negatively impact attempts to address obesity. This article's focus is more on individual and population-based taxation; however, readers interested in corporate responsibility are referred to the many interesting articles and books addressing such in relation to public health and well-being, including, e.g., Wiist 2010 (anti-corporate perspectives).

Ideally, these subsidies would target health-promoting crops;[14] in reality, however, subsidies flow to those crops that many argue contribute to obesity (Fields 2004; Union of Concerned Scientists 2012).

Perhaps more critically, however, in pragmatic terms, the power of taxation might be in its threat, and ensuing prompt for voluntary industry action to avoid government regulation. In the United States, the Clinton Foundation's collaboration with the food and beverage industries, Alliance for a Healthier Generation, is a noteworthy example in its use of voluntary agreements with industry to reduce sugary, high calorie beverage consumption in schools (Clinton Foundation 2012a). Connected to recurring themes, this initiative has focused on targeting children and youth, and also represents a multipronged strategy (Clinton Foundation 2012b). Beyond the United States' shores, concurrent interventions that also include these voluntary approaches have been heralded in recognizing "shared responsibility" between individuals and governments (Federal Ministry 2007; Martin 2008, 5).

Individuals and (Select) Populations: Restricting Access via Purchasing Power & Entitlements

Of course, any tax placed on a food or beverage affects the consumer—as does language like a "fat tax" or "sin tax." Concerns have been raised that these costs are experienced inequitably (Magnusson 2008c; Brownell et al. 2009, 1603; Fletcher, Frisvold, and Tefft 2010; Caraher and Cowburn 2005). Beyond debates over "fat taxes," however, is another potentially divisive approach within the United States: to target users of food stamps (food purchase subsidies for select low-income individuals and families) and limit what they can purchase with such. New York City, the State of Minnesota, and the State of Florida have all sought approval from the USDA to restrict food stamp recipients from using them on "junk foods" (McGeehan 2011; *Los Angeles Times* 2004; Kaczor 2012). All failed, failures that may be read as a result of political lobbying—but deeper still, a distrust in the United States of intrusion on individual liberty (Sullum 2004). And yet, when tailored a certain way, it seems that even the United States is okay with taxing certain behaviors, especially if they can be presented as targeting "them" (rather than "us").

Behavioral Economics and Insurance

"Rewards"

For some time now, U.S. healthcare payers—be they private insurers, government insurers, or employers—have looked for ways to bring down costs of healthcare via insurance-based incentives for "healthy" behaviors. Prominent among approaches are wellness benefits, e.g., discounts on gym memberships and additional rewards for reaching certain targets (e.g., successful weight loss, maintenance of weight, and joining get fit walking campaign). Federal law stands behind these "rewards," by crafting within the Health Insurance Portability and Accountability Act ("HIPAA") a waiver to its anti-discrimination provisions that allow employer rewards to employees, such as premium

---

[14] The World Health Organization highlighted the politically aligned concerns likely to be raised by those who are not thusly subsidized (e.g., certain corn, meat, and dairy producers): that subsidies unfairly influence market conditions (Goodman and Anise 2006, 18).

discounts or waiver of cost-sharing requirements—so long as they are capped at 20% (HIPAA 2009). Effective July 2014, the new ACA legislation raises the cap to 30% (potentially up to 50%) (ACA 2010, § 1201). This means that an individual, say, with a USD$100 premium for a healthcare service, under this wavier, could have it lowered to USD$70 if he/she meet certain targets or follow certain programs.[15]

All of this has been presented as a "reward" on behavior. An individual targeted, however, may experience it as something much different, especially in the face of a new twist on the "wellness incentive." Is it truly a reward, or a surcharge? Is the focus best placed on those given discounts, or those taxed?

Subsidies/"Taxes"

As of January 1, 2010, Alabama became the first state in the United States to impose a surcharge on obese state workers covered by its state insurance plan who do not lose weight (Alabama House Bill 396 2008). Affected state employees with a BMI[16] of 35+ now have one year to lose weight or face an additional USD$25/month surcharge. This expanded an existing surcharge program for smokers. It is worth noting that in 2010, Alabama's obesity rate was 32.2%, the third highest in the United States (behind Mississippi and West Virginia) (CDC 2012a). Interestingly, the "surcharge" was framed as a premium discount: All covered individuals would submit to baseline readings of blood pressure, cholesterol, glucose, and BMI (free screening); those who meet defined targets or engage in healthy behaviors get a USD$25 discount (SEIB 2012). While wellness incentive plans have proven fairly uncontroversial, this is the first instance of expansion of an incentive to a specific risk factor (i.e., BMI) and it has not gone unnoticed.

Next, the State of North Carolina attempted to implement a surcharge approach with its state employees, under the auspices of a new "Comprehensive Wellness Initiative," that would have changed the default plan for state workers to a 70/30 co-insurance plan (North Carolina Senate Bill 287 2009). State workers who did not smoke and had a BMI under 40 or participated in a weight management program could however have qualified for an 80/20 plan (North Carolina Senate Bill 287 2009, sec. 2(a) and 2(b)). As in Alabama, obesity rates and costs were cited factors in this Initiative. In 2010, North Carolina's adult obesity rate was 27.8%—the 21st highest of 50 states (CDC 2012a), with evidence indicating that obesity-related health costs drove up health spending by 37% (North Carolina Senate Bill 287 2009). Notably, in 2011 (shortly before the BMI provisions were to become effective), the "Comprehensive Wellness Initiative" was repealed (North Carolina Session Law 2011-85); thus, Alabama appears to remain alone in its efforts. Yet, other states, too, are watching what is happening in the United States' "laboratory" of states (Mello, Studdert, and Brennan 2006; Fossett et al. 2007). Of interest, a similar surcharge was considered for South Carolina state workers (Chourey 2009), but was dropped and in its place emerged a pilot program to cover gastric bypass and Lap-Band surgery for certain state workers (Wenger 2010). It is not a stretch to expect states across the nation, especially those with high obesity rates, to keep an eye on Alabama and South Carolina.

---

[15] For cautionary remarks on data behind effectiveness of these "rewards," see Volpp et al (2011).

[16] As with BMI reporting by schools, this author did not identify extensive published records evidencing concern over use of BMI as a measure.

Also an attractive "them" to target in the U.S. obesity debate are Medicaid populations. Medicaid is the public-funded healthcare system for primarily low-income individuals, with its initial roots in expanded coverage for individuals and families receiving cash assistance (Kaiser Commission on Medicaid and the Uninsured 2010). Today, it covers one in three children, more than one in three births, one in four poor non-elderly adults, as well as millions of persons with disabilities (Kaiser Family Foundation 2011). A jointly financed program between each individual state and the federal government (with federal government matching state spending on Medicaid), the program includes a mandated list of basic required services, which many states choose to supplement to various degrees with additional services and/or for an expanded pool of individuals and families. In essence, Medicaid is like 50 individual programs (Kaiser Commission on Medicaid and the Uninsured 2010, 5).

In April of 2011, it was reported that the State of Arizona was considering imposing a USD$50/year fee on adult Medicaid patients without children who were obese or smoked (Carlson 2011; Adamy 2011). It was promoted within the state, however, as a way to save USD$500M/year in Medicaid spending plus restore transplantation coverage (cut in 2010) to Medicaid and reduce the number of childless adults not qualifying for Medicaid (Adamy 2011). To do so, the program needed to find cost savings with some other population, and the population thus identified: adults without children, on Medicaid, and who were "fat" or smokers. While Arizona's Proposed Medicaid Reform plan did not end up with this fee under a short-term reform proposal of "personal responsibility" (Arizona Medicaid Reform Plan 2012),[17] it still exists as a potential "longer term reform"—a "wellness effort ... exploring financial penalties for unhealthy behaviors such as smoking and obesity" (Arizona Proposed Medicaid Reform Plan 2012).

The idea of taxing obese persons more is not solely U.S. thinking. In 2010, a member of the German Parliament (from Saxony) argued out of fairness that Germany should hold those who "deliberately lead unhealthy lives ... financially accountable for that" (Collins 2010). While this idea did not become law, a search for ways to restrain healthcare costs experienced by governments and populations suggests what is happening in the United States may be watched by those beyond as well as within its borders. One cautionary note: For countries with a mix of public and private payment (e.g., Australia), there are concerns that taxing certain individuals for "unhealthy" behaviors will push them into public plans, raising public costs (i.e., cost shifting versus cost saving) (Magnusson 2008c).

Japan has taken a different approach: to tax insurers if failing to meet health targets. Notably, as indicated earlier, Japan is not known for having an obesity problem; however, this does not mean its government is not aware of global trends that it hopes to prevent within its shores. And yet, rather than focus on the individual insured, Japan's Healthcare Reform Act of 2006 requires public health insurers to provide health check-ups to beneficiaries ages 40–70, and to craft behavioral interventions to reach government-set targets (International Longevity Center Japan 2008). Beginning in 2013, public insurers face financial penalties for not meeting targets. Japan also shifts costs to the private sector and local governments via the "metabo" law (Onishi 2008; Nakamura 2009). This law, passed in 2008, sets a maximum waistline for employed adults ages 40–74. Employers and local governments are expected to do annual waistline checks and if the maximum is exceeded, counseling must be offered. If the number of overweight

---

[17] Notably, Arizona's Medicaid Reform Plan's request for the annual fee on smokers was not approved by the federal Center for Medicare and Medicaid Services ("CMS") (Arizona Medicaid Reform Plan 2012).

employees is not reduced by 10% in 2012 and 25% in 2015, employers may be required to pay more into the healthcare program for the elderly. While there is some concern that this approach to confront rising healthcare costs may incentivize unhealthy approaches to waistline reduction among employees (especially men) in the period leading up to check-ups (Onishi 2008), it is an interesting shift in responsibility to private actors to keep individual employees healthy. In the political world of obesity, where a government places responsibility or whom it chooses to tax is revealing.

Ultimately, whether any of these more individualized or market-based financial incentives will lead to macro-level cost controls remains to be seen.

"Value-Based" Health Insurance

"What are the treatments that do the most good for the most people at the least amount of cost?" –Jack Friedman, Chief Executive of Providence Health Plans (Appleby 2010)

Despite diverse contexts, nations seemingly converge on this next emerging trend in health coverage: "value-based" insurance design (National Business Coalition on Health 2009). "The basic premise of value-based insurance design is to align out-of-pocket spending with the value of medical services" (Fendrick, Smith and Chernew 2010, 2017).[18] This is nothing new, e.g., for years U.S.-based plans have used tiered coverage systems for pharmacy benefits, with lower co-pays for "preferred" (e.g., generic) prescription medications. Increasingly, however, there are efforts to use financial incentives to steer people away from "low-value" options, and not simply to incentivize doing "high=valued" things (Fendrick, Smith and Chernew 2010; Choudhry, Rosenthal, and Milstein 2010; Robinson 2010; Kapowich 2010). Building on the behavioral economics theory (Orszag 2008; Volpp et al. 2011), financial incentives are seen as an ideal mechanism to accomplish these "value" goals.

"Value-based" insurance design structures may take many forms, e.g., a lower co-pay on medications if participating in a disease management program (Choudhry, Rosenthal, and Milstein, 2010, 1990–1991). Critical for the discussion herein, one can see value-based coverage designs extending to weight management, e.g., incentivize weight loss program participation, regular check-ups, use of approved medications, and the like. States like West Virginia (West Virginia BMS 2009; Bishop and Brodkey 2006), Oregon (Kapowich 2010), and Connecticut (SEBAC 2011; Becker 2011a; Becker 2011b) have taken this next step, targeting Medicaid and state worker populations, tying "valued" actions to regular screenings and appointments, and disease management participation—with financial consequences for non- or failed participation. As one union leader described the result: it is a "nudge" for better care (Becker 2011a). Moreover, the ACA also endorses this "value-based" trend, calling for guidelines that would permit group health plans or health insurance plans to use value-based insurance designs (ACA 2010, § 2713(c)).

---

[18] A separate article will explore the specifics of value-based healthcare and implications for "therapeutic" and evidence-based policymaking.

These "value-based" approaches likely look familiar to nations outside the United States. Most of the nations discussed herein have some governmental body tracking effectiveness and cost-evidence of interventions to promote "value" in evidence-based practices ("EBPs").[19] Collectively, even if advisory, these bodies have some influence on what public and private payers cover, how, and for whom. And inasmuch as they touch upon obesity—what is covered, how and why—they merit a watchful eye, as does who defines "value."

Trends and Themes

Nations seeking to address obesity face a complex interweaving of influences at many levels: individual, family, community, public, industry, cabinet/agency, private and public policy, and regional and transnational trends. Further, government response (or lack thereof) embeds itself in a historical tradition, socio-cultural context, and economic and political environment. Pressure, it seems, comes from all corners. Thus, do we witness a myriad of approaches, targeting individual behavior, public response, corporate responsibility, and/or government role. This part provides but a snapshot of this complexity, from which some trends and themes emerge.

Trends

Within the United States, trends include: use of states as laboratories to test various approaches (and also tailor approaches for localized needs); a disinclination to limit private actors' ability to advertise their products (but offering incentives to voluntarily do so); and use of a market-oriented prism through which to see the individual as consumer who would benefit from the information to make decisions (Mello, Studdert, and Brennan 2006). Beyond the United States, trends seem less driven by individual liberty language and more by a collective responsibility to act, building on welfare state traditions.

Uniting all nations, however, is a critical crosscutting trend: the politics of obesity, which impacts who (e.g., individual, corporation) a government can target and how (e.g., tax, advertising restriction). This, in turn, can set off intense lobbying or pressure by nongovernmental stakeholders against a turn to a "nanny state" (Montopoli 2011; Pandya 2011; Watson 2011). And yet, targeting children is much more politically palatable. So too are efforts to engage industry in voluntary behavior change, and efforts to alter demand via economic incentives. All nations seek to construct a "healthy behavior" ideal, although how it is determined and by whom is much less settled.

Finally, some—as in Japan—are moving beyond "either/or" thinking to what Sugarman and Sandman (2008) have called a "third-way solution" (Sugarman and Sandman 2008, 9): the use of "performance-based regulation" wherein incentives are created for private actors to reach targets, which if not met, allows money (via penalties) to be fed back into the public system. This potentially allows for some consensus among those in the laissez-faire and government mandate camps.

---

[19] Japan is noteworthy, here, for its lack of a body to date to perform or review comparative effectiveness research (Commonwealth Fund 2011, 76).

In sum, all nations situate their use of evidence (what of it exists) in a political context rich with tradition, which informs what they can (even if not "should") do and how. Each faces similar issues: What (if) level of government response is most effective and why? Is it effective generally or only in context? Who bears responsibility to enhance effectiveness and why? Who determines what is effective, and what is "healthy?" And ultimately, who should bear the cost for what is and what could be vis-à-vis obesity/health, and why? The snapshot on how these questions are beginning to be answered, in turn, lead to some themes.

Themes

From the preceding, we see that context matters: the historical, socio-cultural, and political climate all impact whether government assumes a role in addressing obesity, and if so, the type of approach or approaches selected. However, all nations look fundamentally to the data—the number of lives affected (especially children) and costs placed on the public or private system—to help determine the best approach. Some are grounded more in individual liberty and rights of individuals to make choices (but then perhaps pay more for such choices). Here, we might see more individual insured taxes or employer-based subsidies for "wellness"—a more privatized approach. The United States comes to mind with these, although it also endorses certain public health models and population-based efforts, but typically with a voluntary (versus mandated) mindset. Too, other nations are not immune to industry pressures, and also recognize private actors' influence on the issue of obesity and hence need to be part of any solution(s), with greater support for approaches that enhance voluntary action.

Alternatively, especially prominent in Western European nations and Australia, we see government responses based more on a tradition of solidarity, social welfare, or a sense of collective responsibility. Here, we might see more cost shifting across populations versus on specific individuals; however, this does not mean such nations are averse to individual taxes. In fact, most nations discussed herein have at least considered food and beverage taxes that disproportionately impact lower income individuals (with the United States actually more resistant at times, given an often anti-tax, pro-free market political dialogue). As for healthcare taxes/subsidies, perhaps it should not be surprising that publicly funded systems—whether in the United States or, more prominently, in other OECD member nations—are more supportive of "value" approaches in healthcare given greater onus to hold down taxpayer costs in a publicly financed system.

Reflecting on approaches taken, even from a mere snapshot of such, suggests a real tension between individualizing the issue or "public"-izing the issue, and between privatizing and "public"-izing the issue. When the public, via the government, does get involved, a critical theme is that of equity. Are food or beverage taxes regressive (Brownell et al. 2009; Magnusson 2008a, 8)? Do taxes on obese insureds perpetuate inequity on those already marginalized in society (e.g., the poor, racial/ethnic minorities)? A concern is that arguments that tout the benefits to "the system" or "the public" ignore the effects of interventions on the already marginalized (Magnusson 2008b, 7; Volpp et al. 2011).

These equity concerns should not be taken lightly, and building on another theme, they suggest that more evidence (beyond effects on public coffers) is needed to address the impact of given governmental approaches on all stakeholders. While it is pragmatically impossible to wait for "perfect" information, policymakers can at the very least try to be responsible in how they act and also treat their policies as interventions that create new evidence to track and assess (Magnusson 2008c, 7; Campbell 2010).

In sum, in light of all this complexity and unclear evidence base, a strong theme given the tenor of our times is that of incrementalism: "...this is indeed an era that fiercely favors caution, pragmatism, incremental adaptation, voluntarism (not regulation), [and] innovative partnerships.... It is not an era the favors bold transformation" (Morrison 2011).

IV Conclusion and Policy Implications

> "Learning from one another must be the motto." (Federal Ministry 2007)

While simply a snapshot of what is happening in certain industrialized OECD member nations, this review suggests that governments have at their ready a variety of tools to use to try to affect obesity numbers and mechanisms through which to do it. Significantly, this review also suggests there is not a deep amount of data informing option selection and equally critically, the tracking of effectiveness of policy interventions. The key, thus, is expanding the evidence base of what works, when, and how; moreover, we must ascertain who is determining what "effective" means, and seek broader stakeholder input into such if we wish to address equity, and likely long-term effectiveness, concerns.

More importantly for the purposes of this review, any of this testing and talk of effectiveness must pay more attention to the context for proposed and enacted policy interventions: the history informing policy options, the socio-cultural setting in which options would be implemented, and the political traditions and current trends that promote or impede the consideration of certain options. And one cannot ignore the economic climate in which this takes place. Contextual complexity does not imply it is foolhardy to attempt comparative analysis, or to seek ideas from abroad; in fact, it seems more foolhardy not to learn from what others are doing. This emphasis on context serves merely to caution against drawing the wrong conclusions, such as concluding that what works in France, say, will (never) work if adopted in Germany.[20]

And yet, even if "one size does not fit all," comparative investigation highlights promising studies and policy interventions, and the mechanisms assisting in effective travel from evidence generation to policy-based evidence application. Too, comparative investigation that takes serious what undergirds that which is being compared can also elucidate environments that are more or less amenable to given mechanisms for change (Magnusson 2008, 2 online). Collaboration through openness to learning and sharing ideas seems promising, even if creation of templates for wholesale adoption seems unlikely.

If we assume, as this author does, that the government will play some role in the discussion, if only to coalesce discussion (but ideally going beyond that to show true leadership), it seems advisable to be more transparent and accountable up front about

---

[20] For more discussion of the challenges of policy diffusion and adaption across European Union nations, see, e.g., Holzinger and Knill (2005); Knill (2005); Turner and Green (2007); Bulmer (2007).

what that role is—and can be. And the complexity of the issue and context suggests that the answers will not be "do this or that," but rather, "do this and a whole host of that"—a "whole of government" approach (Sacks, Swinburn, and Lawrence 2008, 6; see also Caraher and Cowburn 2005). These contextual considerations of comparative trends and divergences should also be situated within a larger global context. That is, the unit of measurement of analysis does not "simply" rest at the individual, public, or even state, national, or regional level. Rather, added to this should be globalization trends that bond and bind nations, e.g., trade agreements, environmental agreements, and border-transcending bodies such as global corporations (with potential corporate "welfare" policies) and nongovernmental organizations. Thus, this article only hints at the complexity of comparative learning and ability to locally apply "what works" elsewhere. A globalizing world may necessitate a global reaction, including to the issue of obesity. Moreover, given the complexity and morass of actors, policies, and interests, it is not surprising that global attention is sought to harness more resources and political will.

Comparative analysis that contributes to collaborative dialogue can strengthen search for transnational measures of policy effectiveness: Governing bodies may not agree on entry and endpoints, but perhaps they can develop a collective vision of what should be considered when implementing policy interventions (e.g., equity, importance of noneconomic effects of economic approaches). Too, global insights can help flesh out a collectively informed expansion of prisms through which to view policy-level mechanisms for effective change, and more nuanced understanding of what works—therapeutically—as applied in practice (Campbell 2010). These lessons learned and collective measures, then, could feed back into intra-national discussions.

Next Steps

To render the discussion concrete, what might be helpful next steps? Urged, as noted above, is openness to meaningful engagement with other nation's policymakers to learn from successes and failures, and better identify facilitators and barriers, to effective obesity prevention. Critically, this must take place with a much more studied, systematic review of the various contexts for policy-level obesity action. The latter might also suggest a next step of data collection: While the evidence base is growing for interventions to address obesity, less is known about what policies facilitate these evidence-based approaches.

Inserting policy as a critical implementation lever in the translation of research to practice, and then studying what policies are most effective in achieving sought ends (as mutually understood and clearly defined), is critical to achieve the sort of global work envisioned herein. Specifically pictured is development of a "map" of what works, where, how, and with what support—at local, state, regional, national, and transnational levels. This research and mapping can, in turn, feature for policymakers where policy environments are more effective than others in addressing obesity and at what costs, to enhance (ideally) more evidence-based policymaking. Humility, added to openness to learning, added to commitment to data tracking and quality improvement might thus add flesh to calls to action to address obesity. And, as this article's snapshot highlights, it is imperative not to ignore the context within which these activities take place, and how context impacts the policymaking process and resultant policies—thus a critical variable for any comparative (and internal) analysis.

In sum, policymaking has consequences; when the government acts (and accepting the current status quo is in essence an "action"), lives are affected. So, by learning from one another policymakers can better illuminate and then examine those consequences with a more robust set of data points to compare, and eyes with which to do the comparison. In light of the growing numbers affected by obesity—in human and economic terms—ideally governments would act with more vision of what informs their action, e.g., the state of the evidence (as generated by whom) and the context in which that evidence is accepted, modified, or discarded. And so, there is value in comparative investigation—if simply to acknowledge the complexity and add more voices to the discussion of effective next steps to confront obesity in a diverse but interconnected global society.

References

About-france.com. 2012. "The French Political System." http://about-france.com/political-system.htm (accessed March 30, 2012).

ACA. 2010. Public Law 111-148. Section 1201. PHSA Sec. 2705.

Adamy, J. 2011. "Arizona Proposes Medicaid Fat Fee." WSJ.com. April 1, 2011. http://online.wsj.com/article/SB10001424052748704530204576235151262336300.html (accessed March 29, 2012).

Administrative Management Bureau. 2007. "Fundamental Structure of the Government of Japan." Ministry of Internal Affairs and Communications. http://www.kantei.go.jp/foreign/constitution_and_government_of_japan/fundamental_e.html (accessed March 30, 2012).

Alabama House Bill. 2008. Public Act No. 2008-280 (2008, enacted, AL HB 396).

Appleby, J. 2010. "Insurers Test Health Plans that Stress Patient Choices." *USA Today*. March 11, 2010. [Online].
http://www.usatoday.com/money/industries/health/2010-03-11-valuehealthcare11_CV_N.htm (accessed March 29, 2012).

Arizona Medicaid Reform Plan. 2012. Section B.6. "Personal Responsibility Reforms SAHCCCS Activities." updated January 18, 2012.

Arizona Proposed Medicaid Reform Plan, page 5. azgovernor.gov/dms/upload/PR_031511_AHCCCSSummary.pdf (accessed March 29, 2012).

Arkansas Act 1220. 2003. State of Arkansas, 84th General Assembly Regular Session.

Allais, O., P. Bertail, and V. Nichèle. 2010. "The Effects of a Fat Tax on FrenchHouseholds' Purchases: A Nutritional Approach." *American Journal of Agricultural Economics* 92 (1): 228-245.

Australian Bureau of Statistics. 2007. "20680-Country of Birth of Person (minor groups) by Sex-Australia."
http://www.censusdata.abs.gov.au/ABSNavigation/prenav/ViewData?breadcrumb=POLTD&method=Place%20of%20Usual%20Residence&subaction=-1&issue=2006&producttype=Census%20Tables&documentproductno=0&textversion=false&documenttype=Details&collection=Census&javascript=true&topic=Birthplace&action=404&productlabel=Country%20of%20Birth%20of%20Person%20%28minor%20groups%29%20by%20Sex&order=1&period=2006&tabname=Details&areacode=0&navmapdisplayed=true& (accessed June 1, 2012).

Australian Bureau of Statistics. 2010. "3201.0—Population by Age and Sex, Australian States and Territories, Jun 2010."
http://www.abs.gov.au/ausstats/abs@.nsf/mf/3201.0 (accessed March 30, 2012).

Australian Bureau of Statistics. 2011. "Overweight and Obesity in Adults in Australia: A Snapshot." National Health Survey 2007-08, Pub. No. 4842.0.55.001. http://www.abs.gov.au/AUSSTATS/abs@.nsf/DetailsPage/4842.0.55.0012007%E2%80%9308 (accessed March 29, 2012).

Australian Government. 2008a. "Overweight and Obesity in Australia." http://www.health.gov.au/internet/healthyactive/publishing.nsf/Content/overweight-obesity (accessed March 27, 2012).

Australian Government. 2008b. "Obesity in Australia." http://www.health.gov.au/internet/preventativehealth/publishing.nsf/Content/E233F8695 823F16CCA2574DD00818E64/$File/obesity-2.pdf (accessed March 27, 2012).

Australian Government. 2012a. "Germany Country Brief." Department of Foreign Affairs and Trade. http://www.dfat.gov.au/geo/germany/ germany_brief.html (accessed March 30, 2012).

Australian Government. 2012b. "Denmark Country Brief." Department of Foreign Affairs and Trade. http://www.dfat.gov.au/geo/denmark/ denmark_brief.html (accessed March 30, 2012).

Australian Government. 2012c. "Australia's System of Government." Department of Foreign Affairs and Trade. http://www.dfat.gov.au /facts/sys_gov.html (accessed March 30, 2012).

BBC. 2012." Languages Across Europe." http://www.bbc.co.uk/ languages/european_languages/countries/uk.shtml (accessed March 30, 2012).

BBC News. 2011. "Denmark Introduces World's First Food Fat Tax." October 1, 2011. [Online]. http://www.bbc.co.uk/news/world-europe-15137948 (accessed March 29, 2012).

Becker, A.L. 2011a. "Shift to Value-Based Health Plan Can Cause Worker Anxiety." The CT Mirror [Online], June 2, 2011. http://www.ctmirror.org/story/12788/value-based-health-plan (accessed March 29, 2012).

Becker, A.L. 2011b. "Health Care Deal could Save Money, but Skeptics Question How Soon." The CT Mirror [Online], May 20, 2011. http://ctmirror.org/story/12663/health-care-deal-could-produce-savings-skeptics-question-how-fast (accessed March 29, 2012).

Berger J. 2010. "New Strategy for Soda Tax Gives Diet Drinks a Break." *The New York Times*, May 19, 2010. [Online] http://www.nytimes.com/2010/05/20/nyregion/20sodatax.html?_r=2 (accessed March 29, 2012).

Bishop, G., and A.C. Brodkey. 2006. "Personal Responsibility and Physician Responsibility—West Virginia's Medicaid Plan." *New England Journal of Medicine* 355 (8): 756-758.

Boomgaarden, H., R. Andreas, M. Schuck, and C. Vreese. 2011. "Mapping EU Attitudes: Conceptual and Empirical Dimensions of Euroscepticism and EU Support." *European Union Politics* 12 (2): 241-266.

Boozman College of Public Health. 2009. "Year Five Evaluation: Arkansas Act 1220 of 2003 to Combat Childhood Obesity." University of Arkansas for Medical Sciences. http://www.rwjf.org/pr/product.jsp?id=41069 (accessed March 29, 2012).

Brownell, K., T. Farley, W. Willett, B. Popkin, F. Chaloupka, J. Thompson, and D. Ludwig. 2009. "The Public Health and Economic Benefits of Taxing Sugar-Sweetened Beverages." *The New England Journal of Medicine* 361 (16): 1599-1605.

Buffery, V. 2011. "French VAT Hike to Hit Pizzas, Quiches—not Baguettes." Reuters. 29 December. http://www.reuters.com/article/2011/ 12/29/us-france-vat-idUSTRE7BS12R20111229?feedType=RSS&feedName= lifestyleMolt (accessed March 29, 2012).

Bulmer, S. 2007. "Britain and the European Union: Convergence through Policy Transfer?" *German Politics* 16 (1): 39-57.

Campbell, A.T. 2010. "Therapeutic Jurisprudence: A Framework for Evidence-Informed Health Care Policymaking." *International Journal of Law and Psychiatry* 233: 281-292.

Campbell, A.T. 2012. "Using Therapeutic Jurisprudence to Frame the Role of Emotion in Health Policymaking." *Phoenix Law Review* 5(4): Phoenix Law Review 2012; 5(4): 676-704.

Caraher, M., and G. Cowburn.2005. "Taxing Food: Implications for Public Health Nutrition." *Public Health Nutrition* 8 (8): 1242-1249.

Carlson, M. 2011. "Medicaid Considers Tax on Smokers, Obese." ABCNews [Online]. April 1, 2011. http://abcnews.go.com/Health/wireStory?id=13276359#.T3UMl4XgOkZ (accessed March 29, 2012).

CDC. 2012a. "U.S. Obesity Trends." http://www.cdc.gov/obesity/ data/trends.html (accessed March 26, 2012).

CDC. 2012b. "Health Consequences." http://www.cdc.gov/obesity/causes/health.html (accessed March 26, 2012).

CDC. 2012c. "Economic Consequences." http://www.cdc.gov/obesity/causes/economics.html (accessed March 26, 2012).

CDC. 2012d. "Defining Overweight and Obesity." http://www.cdc.gov/obesity/defining.html (accessed March 26, 2012).

CDC. 2012f. "Obesity and Overweight." http://www.cdc.gov/nchs/fastats/overwt.htm (accessed March 26, 2012).

Central Intelligence Agency. 2012. "The World Factbook." https://www.cia.gov/library/publications/the-world-factbook/ (accessed March 30, 2012).

Choudhry, N., M. Rosenthal, and A. Milstein, 2010. "Assessing the Evidence for Value-Based Insurance Design." *Health Affairs* 29 (11): 1988-1994.

Chourey, S. 2009. "Ryberg Bill wants Obese to Pay More." *The Augusta Chronicle.* January 12, 2009. [Online]. http://chronicle.augusta.com/stories/2009/01/12/met_507328.shtml (accessed March 29, 2012).

Clinton Foundation. 2012a. "Alliance for a Healthier Generation: Industry Initiatives." http://www.clintonfoundation.org/what-we-do/alliance-for-a-healthier-generation/our-approach/industry-initiative (accessed February 20, 2012).

Clinton Foundation. 2012b. "Alliance for a Healthier Generation: Healthy Schools." http://www.clintonfoundation.org/what-we-do/alliance-for-a-healthier-generation/our-approach/healthy-schools-program (accessed February 20, 2012).

Collins H. 2010. "Germany Weighs Tax on the Obese." AOL News [Online]. July 23, 2010. http://www.aolnews.com/2010/07/23/germany-weighs-tax-on-the-obese/ (accessed March 27, 2012).

Commonwealth Fund. 2011. "International Profiles of Health Care Systems, 2011." Commonwealth Fund Publication Number 1562: 113.

Congressional Research Service (CRS). 2001. "American National Government: An Overview." Order Code RS20443. January 22.

Conis, E. 2010. "Mandating Body Mass Index Reporting in the Schools." *Health Policy Monitor* April: 1–6 [Online]. http://www.hpm.org/survey/us/a15/2 (accessed March 29, 2012).

Considine, M. 2002. "Making Up the Government's Mind: Agenda Setting in a Parliamentary System." *Governance: International Journal of Policy, Administration, and Institutions* 11 (3): 297-317.

Cousins, M. 2005. *European Welfare States.* London: Sage Publications.

Darlington, R. 2012. "A Short Guide to the British Political System." February 22. http://rogerdarlington.me.uk/Britishpoliticalsystem.html (accessed March 30, 2012).

De Schutter, O. 2011. "Report Submitted by the Special Rapporteur on the right to food." December 26.

Denmark.dk. 2012. "Government & Politics." http://www.denmark.dk/en/menu/About-Denmark/Government-Politics/ (accessed March 30, 2012).

Direct.gov. 2012a. "Overview of the UK System of Government." http://www.direct.gov.uk/en/Governmentcitizensandrights/UKgovernment/Centralgovern mentandthemonarchy/DG_073438 (accessed March 30, 2012).

Direct.gov. 2012b. "The Government, Prime Minister and Cabinet." http://www.direct.gov.uk/en/Governmentcitizensandrights/UKgovernment/Centralgovern mentandthemonarchy/DG_073444 (accessed March 30, 2012).

Dumanovsky, T., C. Huang, C. Nonas, T. Matte, M. Bassett, and L. Silver, 2011. "Changes in Energy Content of Lunchtime Purchases from Fast Food Restaurants after Introduction of Calorie Labeling: Cross Sectional Customer Surveys." *British Medical Journal* 343: d4464.

Elbel, B., R. Kersh, V. Brescoll, and B. Dixon. 2009. "Calorie Labeling and Food Choices: A First Look at the Effects on Low-Income People in New York City." *Health Affairs* 28 (6): w1110-w1121.

Etzioni, A. 2010a. "Obesity Prevention: A Responsive Communitarian Approach (Part 1)". Health Affairs Blog. July 1, 2010. http://healthaffairs.org/blog/2010/07/01/obesity-prevention-a-responsive-communitarian-approach-part-1/ (accessed March 29, 2012).

Etzioni, A. 2010b. "Obesity Prevention: A Responsive Communitarian Approach (Part 2)." Health Affairs Blog. July 2, 2010. http://healthaffairs.org/blog/2010/07/02/obesity-prevention-a-responsive-communitarian-approach-part-2/ (accessed March 29, 2012).

European Commission. 2006. "Europeans and their Languages." http://ec.europa.eu/public_opinion/archives/ebs/ebs_243_en.pdf (accessed March 30, 2012).

European Commission/Eurostat. 2011. "File: Percentage of Population Aged 65 Years and Over on 1 January of Selected Years." http://epp.eurostat.ec.europa.eu/statistics_explained/index.php?title=File:Percentage_of_ population_aged_65_years_and_over_on_1_January_of_selected_years.PNG&filetimest amp=20110609134420 (accessed March 30, 2012).

Evans, E.W., and K.R. Sonneville, 2009. "BMI Report Cards: Will They Pass or Fail in the Fight Against Pediatric Obesity?" *Current Opinions in Pediatrics* 21: 431-436.

Falleti, T. and J. Lynch, 2009. "Context and Causal Mechanisms in Political Analysis." *Comparative Political Studies* 42 (9): 1143-1166.

Federal Ministry. 2007. "The 'Badenweiler Declaration' " http://www.bmelv.de/SharedDocs/Standardartikel/EN/Food/BadenweilerDeclaration.htm l (accessed March 29, 2012).

Fendrick, A.M., D.G. Smith, and M.E. Chernew. 2010. "Applying Value-Based Insurance Design to Low-Value Health Services." *Health Affairs* 29 (11): 2017-2021.

Fields, S. 2004. "The Fat of the Land: Agricultural Subsidies Foster Poor Health?" *Environment Health Perspectives* 112 (14): A820-A823.

Finkelstein, E., J.G. Trogdon, J.W. Cohen, and W. Dietz. 2009. "Annual Medical Spending Attributable to Obesity: Payer-And Service-Specific Estimates." *Health Affairs* 28 (5): W822-W831.

Finkelstein, E., M. DiBonaventura, S. Burgess, and B. Hale. 2010. "The Cost of Obesity in the Workplace." *Journal of Occupational & Environmental Medicine* 52 (10): 971-976.

Fossett, J., A. Ouellette, S. Philpott, D. Magnus, and G. McGee. 2007. "Federalism & Bioethics: States and Moral Pluralism." *The Hastings Center Report* 37 (6): 24-35.

Fletcher, J., D. Frisvold, and N. Tefft. 2010. "Taxing Soft Drinks and Restricting Access to Vending Machines to Curb Child Obesity." *Health Affairs* 29 (5): 1059-1066.

Gallup Politics. 2011. "Democratic Party ID Drops in 2010, Tying 22-Year Low." January 5. http://www.gallup.com/poll/145463/democratic-party-drops-2010-tying-year-low.aspxow.aspx (accessed March 30, 2012).

Germany.co.za. 2012. "Politics." http://www.germany.co.za/politics.html (accessed March 30, 2012).

Goddard, M., K. Hauck, A. Preker, and P. Smith. 2006. "Priority Setting in Health—a Political Economy Perspective." *Health Economics, Policy and Law* 1: 79-90.

Goodman, C. and A. Anise. 2006. *What is Known about the Effectiveness of Economic Instruments to Reduce Consumption of Foods High in Saturated Fats and other Energy-Dense Foods for Preventing and Treating Obesity?* Copenhagen: WHO Regional Office for Europe. http://www.euro.who.int/document/e88909.pdf (accessed March 29, 2012).

Gostin, L. P. Arno, and A. Brandt. 1997. "FDA Regulation of Tobacco Advertising and Youth Smoking: Historical, Social, and Constitutional Perspectives." *Journal of the American Medical Association* 277 (5): 410-418.

Gostin, L. 2000. "Public Health Law in a New Century." *Journal of the American Medical Association* 283 (23): 3118-3122.

Gostin, L. 2008. *Public Health Law: Power, Duty, Restraint.* Berkeley, CA: University of California Press.

Handsley, E., K. Mehta, J. Coveney, and C. Nehmy. 2009. "Regulatory Axes on Food Advertising to Children on Television." *Australia and New Zealand Health Policy* 6: online.

Hartocollis, A. 2010. "Failure of State Soda Tax Plan Reflects Power of an Antitax Message." July 2, 2010. http://www.nytimes.com/2010/07/03/nyregion/03sodatax.html?pagewanted=all (accessed March 29, 2012).

Harvard School of Public Health. 2012. "Economic Costs of Overweight and Obesity." http://www.hsph.harvard.edu/obesity-program/resources/obesity-economic-cost/index.html (accessed March 29, 2012).

HIPAA. 2009. 45 C.F.R. §146.121(f)(2). 21 Federal Register 75046, December 13, 2006, as amended at 74 Federal Register 51688, October 7, 2009.

Hodge, J., A. Garcia, and S. Shah,. 2008. "Legal Themes Concerning Obesity Regulation in the United States: Theory and Practice." *Australia and New Zealand Health Policy* 5: 14.

Holzinger, K., and C. Knill. 2005. "Causes and Conditions of Cross-National Policy Convergence." *Journal of European Public Policy* 12 (5): 775-796.

International Longevity Center Japan. 2008. "Expanding Health Promotion Efforts: The National Health Insurers begin Conducting Annual Health Checks of all 40–70 year olds in April 2008." http://longevity.ilcjapan.org/t_stories/0801.html (accessed March 29, 2012).

IASO. 2006. "The Sydney Principles." http://www.iaso.org/iotf/obesity/childhoodobesity/sydneyprinciples/ (accessed March 28, 2012).

IASO. 2012. "Marketing to Children." http://www.iaso.org/policy/marketing-children/ (accessed March 29, 2012).

index mundi. 2012. "Germany Demographics Profile 2012." http://www.indexmundi.com/germany/demographics_profile.html (accessed March 30, 2012).

Kaczor, B. 2012. "Bill with Junk Food Ban for Food Stamp Recipients Dies in Florida House." CBS News [Online], February 13, 2012. http://tampa.cbslocal.com/2012/02/13/bill-with-junk-food-ban-for-food-stamp-recipients-dies-in-florida-house/ (accessed March 29, 2012).

Kaiser Commission on Medicaid and the Uninsured. 2010. "Medicaid: A Primer." June. Publication No. 7334-04. http://www.kff.org/medicaid/7334.cfm (accessed June 1, 2012).

Kaiser Family Foundation. "Medicaid Matters: Understanding Medicaid's Role in Our Health Care System." March. Publication #8165. http://www.kff.org (accessed May 1, 2012).

Kaplan, K. 2011. "Fat Tax in Denmark: Why they Have it; Could it Happen in U.S.?" *Los Angeles Times*. October 3, 2011. http://articles.latimes.com/2011/oct/03/news/la-heb-fat-tax-denmark-20111013 (accessed March 29, 2012).

Kapowich, J. 2010. "Oregon's Test of Value-Based Insurance Design in Coverage for State Workers." *Health Affairs* 29 (11): 2028-2032.

Katrandjian, O. 2011. "Denmark Introduces 'Fat Tax' on Foods High in Saturated Fat." ABC News Blog. October 2, 2011. http://abcnews.go.com/blogs/health/2011/10/02/denmark-introduces-fat-tax-on-foods-high-in-saturated-fat/ (accessed March 29, 2012).

Knill, C. 2005. "Introduction: Cross-National Policy Convergence: Concepts, Approaches, and Explanatory Factors." *Journal of European Public Policy* 12 (5): 1-11.

Koplan, J., C. Leverman, and V. Kraak, 2005. *Preventing Childhood Obesity: Health in the Balance*. Washington, DC: National Academies Press.

Los Angeles Times. 2004. "USDA Rejects Ban on Buying Junk Food with Food Stamps." May 8, 2004. [Online]. http://articles.latimes.com/2004/ may/08/nation/na-junkfood8 (accessed March 29, 2012).

Lubbers, M., and P. Scheepers. 2010. "Divergent Trends of Euroscepticism in Countries and Regions of the European Union." *European Journal of Political Research* 49 (6): 787-817.

Lustig, R., L. Schmidt, and C. Brindis. 2012. "The Toxic Truth about Sugar." *Nature* 282: 27-29.

Magnusson, R. 2008a. "Obesity: Should There be a Law Against It? Introduction to a Symposium." *Australia and New Zealand Health Policy* 5: online.

Magnusson, R. 2008b. "What's Law Got to do With it? Part 1: A Framework for Obesity Prevention." *Australia and New Zealand Health Policy* 5: online.

Magnusson, R. 2008c. "What's Law Got to do With it? Part 2: Legal Strategies for Healthier Nutrition and Obesity Prevention." *Australia and New Zealand Health Policy* 5: online.

Martin, R. 2008. "The Role of Law in the Control of Obesity in England: Looking at the Contribution of Law to a Healthy Food Culture." *Australia and New Zealand Health Policy* 5: online.

Masaru, K. 1997. *Japan's Postwar Party Politics.* Princeton: Princeton University Press.

McGeehan, P. 2011. "U.S. Rejects Mayor's Plan to Ban Use of Food Stamps to Buy Soda." *New York Times*, August 19, 2011. http://www.nytimes.com/2011/08/20/nyregion/ban-on-using-food-stamps-to-buy-soda-rejected-by-usda.html (accessed March 29, 2012).

Mello, M., D. Studdert, and T. Brennan, 2006. "Obesity: The New Frontier of Public Health Law." *New England Journal of Medicine* 354 (24): 2601-2610.

Ministére des Affaires Ètrangéres. 2008. "Introduction, the French Political System." http://www.diplomatie.gouv.fr/en/france/institutions-and-politics/the-french-political-system/ (accessed March 30, 2012).

Ministére des Affaires Ètrangéres et Européennes. 2008. "La France a la loupe: Population Trends in France." http://www.ambafrance-eau.org/IMG/Population_trends.pdf (accessed March 30, 2012).

Ministry of Internal Affairs and Communication. 2008. Statistics Bureau, Director-General for Policy Planning. "Chapter 2 Population." http://www.stat.go.jp/english/data/handbook/c02cont.htm (accessed March 30, 2012).

Morrison, J.S. 2011. "NCDs Trigger a Different Model of Response." Center for Strategic & International Studies (CSIS) Publication. September 27, 2011. http://csis.org/publication/ncds-trigger-different-model-response (accessed March 29, 2012).

Montopoli, B. 2011. "GOP decries 'nanny state' Push on Junk Food Ads." CBS News [Online], July 7, 2011. http://www.cbsnews.com/8301-503544_162-20077584-503544.html (accessed March 30, 2012).

Nakamura, D. 2009. "Fat in Japan? You're breaking the law." Global Post, November 10, 2009. [Online]. http://www.globalpost.com/dispatch/ japan/091109/fat-japan-youre-breaking-the-law (accessed March 27, 2012).

National Business Coalition on Health. 2009. *Value-Based Benefit Design: A Purchaser's Guide.* Washington, DC: National Business Coalition on Health.

Nestle, M. 2010. "Health Care Reform in Action—Calorie Labeling Goes National." *New Journal of Medicine* 362: 2343-2345.

Neto, O.A.; and Samuels, D. 2010. "Democratic Regimes and Cabinet Politics: A Global Perspective." *RIEL-Revista Ibero-Americana De Estudos Legislativos* 1 (1): 10-23.

North Carolina Senate Bill 287. 2009. North Carolina Session 2009.

North Carolina Session Law 2011-85. 2011. North Carolina Session 2011, Senate Bill 323.

OECD. 2012a. "Obesity Update 2012." http://www.oecd.org/dataoecd/1/61/49716427.pdf (accessed March 26, 2012).

OECD. 2012b. "Obesity and the Economics of Prevention: Fit not Fat—United States Key Facts." http://www.oecd.org/document/57/0,3746,en_2649_33929_46038969_1_1_1_1,00.html (accessed March 27, 2012).

OECD. 2012c. "Obesity and the Economics of Prevention: Fit not Fat—France Key Facts." http://www.oecd.org/document/26/0,3746,en_2649_ 33929_46038682_1_1_1_1,00.html

Ofcom. 2007. "Television Advertising of Food and Drink Products to Children." February 22, 2007, Final statement.

Onishi, N. 2008. "Japan Seeking Trim Waists, Measures Millions." *The New York Times*, June 13, 2008. [Online]. http://www.nytimes.com/ 2008/06/13/world/asia/13fat.html?pagewanted=all (accessed March 29, 2012).

Orszag, P. 2008. "Health Care and Behavioral Economics: A Presentation to the National Academy of Social Insurance." May 29, 2008. Congressional Budget Office (CBO) Publication 41702. http://cbo.gov/publication/41702 (accessed June 1, 2012).

Parliament of Australia. 2011. "Parliament: An Overview." February 28. http://www.aph.gov.au/parl.htm (accessed March 30, 2012).

Parmet, W. 2008. *Populations, Public Health, and the Law*. Washington, DC: Georgetown University Press.

Pandya, A. 2011. "Watch Out If You are Fat: the EU is on to You." *Daily Mail* [Online]. October 18, 2011. http://www.dailymail.co.uk/debate/article-2050496/Anti-obesity-laws-Watch-fat-EU-you.html (accessed March 30, 2012).

Pomeranz, J. and L. Gostin. 2009. "Improving Laws and Legal Authorities for Obesity Prevention and Control." *Journal of Law, Medicine & Ethics* 37: 62-75.

Powell, L. and F. Chaloupka. 2009. "Food Prices and Obesity: Evidence and Policy Implications for Taxes and Subsidies." *Milbank Quarterly* 87 (1): 229-257.

Puhl, R.M. and C.A. Heuer, 2010. "Obesity Stigma: Important Considerations for Public Health." *American Journal of Public Health* 100 (6): 1019-1028.

Robinson, J. 2010. "Applying Value-Based Insurance Design to High-Cost Services." *Health Affairs* 29 (11): 2009-2016.

Rothman, K. 2008. "BMI-related Errors in the Measurement of Obesity." *International Journal of Obesity* 32: S56-S59.

Ryan, K., P. Higginson, S. McCarthy, M. Justus, and J. Thompson. 2006. "Arkansas Fights Fat: Translating Research into Policy to Combat Childhood and Adolescent Obesity." *Health Affairs* 25 (4): 992-1004.

Sacks, G., Boyd Swinburn, and Mark Lawrence. 2008. "A Systematic Policy approach to Changing the Food System and Physical Activity Environments to Prevent Obesity." *Australia and New Zealand Health Policy* 5: 13.

Schoen, C. R. Osborn, D. Squires, M. Doty, R. Pierson, and S. Applebaum, 2010. "How Health Insurance Design Affects Access to Care and Costs, by Income, in Eleven Countries." *Health Affairs* Web First, November 18, 2010.

School Directory. 2012. "The Languages Spoken in Japan." http://www.spainexchange.com/guide/JP-language.htm (accessed March 30, 2012).

SEBAC. 2011. Agreement between State of Connecticut and State Employees Bargaining Agent Coalition (SEBAC), Section IIA2 (Health Enhancement Program) and Attachment B. May 27, 2011.

SEIB. 2012. "Wellness Program." https://www.alseib.org/ HealthInsurance/SEHIP/Wellness.aspx (accessed March 29, 2012).

Shah, N.R., and E.R. Braverman. 2012. "Measuring Adiposity in Patients: The Utility of Body Mass Index (BMI), Percent Body Fat, and Leptin." *PLoS ONE* 7(4): e33308. doi:10.1371/journal.pone.0033308

Shugart, M. 1993. "Of Presidents and Parliaments." 2 1 *East European Constitutional Review*: 30 - 32.

Smith, T., B. Lin, and L. Lee. 2010. "Taxing Caloric Sweetened Beverages: Potential Effects on Beverage Consumption, Calorie Intake, and Obesity." U.S. Department of Agriculture, Economic Research Service. Economic Research Report No. 100. Sorenson, C. "Love Me, Love Me Not... A Typology of Public Euroscepticism." SEI Working Paper No. 101, EPERN Working Paper No. 19, January 2008. http://www.sussex.ac.uk/sei/research/europeanpartieselectionsreferendumsnetwork/epern workingpapers (accessed March 29, 2012).

Spiegel Online International. 2007. "Germans Are Fattest People in Europe, Study Shows." [Online]. http://www.spiegel.de/international/europe/ 0,1518,478303,00.html (accessed March 27, 2012).

State of Hawaii, Department of Taxation. 2000. "General Excise vs. Sales Tax." Tax Facts 96-1.

Sugarman S.D., N. Sandman. 2008. "Using Performance-Based Regulation to Reduce Childhood Obesity," *Australia and New Zealand Heatlh Policy* 5: online.

Sullum, J. 2004. "The War on Fat." *Reason Magazine* [Online]. http://reason.com/archives/2004/08/01/the-war-on-fat (accessed March 29, 2012).

Swinburn, B. 2008. "Obesity Prevention: the Role of Policies, Laws and Regulations." *Australia and New Zealand Health Policy* 5: 12.

Swinburn B., G. Egger, and F. Raza. "Dissecting Obesogenic Environments: The Development and Application of a Framework for Identifying and Prioritizing Environmental Interventions for Obesity." *Preventive Medicine* Dec; 29 (6 Pt. 1): 563-570.

Thaler, R. and C. Sunstein, 2008. *Nudge: Improving Decisions about Health, Wealth, and Happiness.* Yale University Press: New Haven, CT.

The Economist. 2008. "France: Political Structure." September 26. http://www.economist.com/node/12282906 (accessed March 30, 2012).

The Local. 2010. "Teachers Call for Student Weigh-ins to Curb Obesity." DDP/The Local, June 4, 2010. [Online]. http://www.thelocal.de/ national/20100604-27643.html (accessed March 29, 2012).

The Telegraph. 2011. "Conservative Party Conference 2011: Fat Tax Could Be Introduced in Britain." October 4, 2011. [Online]. http://www.telegraph.co.uk/news/politics/conservative/8806350/Conservative-Party-Conference-2011-fat-tax-could-be-introduced-in-Britain.html (accessed March 26, 2012).

Turner, E.; and Green, S. 2007. "Understanding Policy Convergence in Britain and Germany. *German Politics* 16 (1): 1-21.

U.K. National Statistics. 2012. "Topic guide to: Older People." http://www.statistics.gov.uk/hub/population/ageing/older-people (March 30, 2012).

United Nations (UN). 2011. "2011 High Level Meeting on Prevention and Control of Non-communicable diseases." http://www.un.org/en/ga/ncdmeeting2011/ (March 29, 2012).

Unicef. 2012a. "United Kingdom, Statistics." http://www.unicef.org/infobycountry/uk_statistics.html (accessed March 30, 2012).

Unicef. 2012b. "France, Statistics." http://www.unicef.org/infobycountry/france_statistics.html (accessed March 30, 2012).

Unicef. 2012c. "Germany, Statistics." http://www.unicef.org/infobycountry/germany_statistics.html (accessed March 30, 2012).

Unicef. 2012d. "Denmark, Statistics." http://www.unicef.org/infobycountry/denmark_statistics.html (accessed March 30, 2012).

Unicef. 2012e. "Australia, Statistics."http://www.unicef.org/infobycountry/australia_statistics.html (accessed March 30, 2012).

Unicef. 2012f. "Japan, Statistics."http://www.unicef.org/infobycountry/japan_statistics.html (accessed March 30, 2012).

U.S. Census Bureau. 2010. "Language Spoken at Home." http://factfinder2.census.gov/faces/tableservices/jsf/pages/productview.xhtml?pid=ACS_10_1YR_S1601&prodType=table (accessed March 30, 2012).

U.S. Census Bureau. 2011a. "Overview of Race and Hispanic Origin: 2010." 2010 Census Briefs: Census Briefs: C2010BR-02. March.

U.S. Census Bureau. 2011b. "Age and Sex Composition: 2010." 2010 Census Brief: Report c2010br-03.

U.S. Census Bureau. 2012. "State & County QuickFacts: USA." http://quickfacts.census.gov/qfd/states/00000.html (accessed March 30, 2012).

U.S. Department of State. 2011a. "Background Note: Japan." August 23. http://www.state.gov/r/pa/ei/bgn/4142.htm (accessed March 30, 2012).

U.S. Department of State. 2011b. "July-December, 2010 International Religious Freedom Report." http://www.state.gov/j/drl/rls/irf/2010_5/index.htm (accessed March 30, 2012).

USA Today. 2009. "Rising Obesity will Cost U.S. Health Care $344 billion a Year." November 17, 2009. [Online]. http://www.usatoday.com/news/health/weightloss/2009-11-17-future-obesity-costs_N.htm (accessed March 27, 2012).

USA Today. 2011. "Philly Council Weighing Soda Tax." June 16, 2011. [Online]. http://yourlife.usatoday.com/parenting-family/story/2011/06/Philly-Council-weighing-soda-tax/48496688/1 (accessed March 29, 2012).

Union of Concerned Scientists. 2012. "Toward Healthy Foods and Farms: How Science-Based Policies Can Transform Agriculture." Policy Brief. http://www.ucsusa.org/food_and_agriculture/solutions/big_picture_solutions/healthy-food-and-farms-policy.html (accessed March 29, 2012).

Volpp, K.G., D.A. Asch, R. Galvin, and G. Lowenstein. 2011. "Redesigning Employee Health Incentives—Lessons from Behavioral Economics." *New England Journal of Medicine* 365 (5): 388-390.

Washington Post. 1998. "Major Political Parties in Japan." http://www.washingtonpost.com/wp-srv/inatl/longterm/japan/japanparties.htm (accessed March 30, 2012).

Watson, D. 2011. "The Nanny State's New Food Frontier." Business Spectator. December 9, 2011. [Online] http://www.businessspectator.com.au/bs.nsf/Article/food-industry-tobacco-health-Australia-Canberra-go-pd20111209-PD3BK?OpenDocument&src=is&cat=food%20_%20beverages-al (accessed March 30, 2012).

Watson, L. 2011. "France Approves Fat Tax on Sugary Drinks such as Coca-Cola and Fanta." *Daily Mail* [Online]. 29 December 2011. http://www.dailymail.co.uk/news/article-2079796/France-approves-fat-tax-sugary-drinks-Coca-Cola-Fanta.html (accessed March 29, 2012).

Web Japan. 2012. "Governmental Structure." http://web-japan.org/ (accessed March 30, 2012).

Wenger, Y. 2010. "State to Pay for Bariatric Surgeries." The Post and Courier. August 13, 2010. [Online]. http://postandcourier.com/article/20100813/PC1602/308139934 (accessed March 29, 2012).

West Virginia Bureau of Medicaid Services (BMS). 2009. *BMS Manual: Chapter 527 Covered Services, Limitations, and Exclusions for Mountain Health Choices.* Section 527.4.2 (Promoting Member Choice and Responsibility) and Appendix 2. January 30. http://www.dhhr.wv.gov/bms/ mhc/Pages/default.aspx (accessed March 29, 2012).

Wiist, W.H., ed. 2010. *The Bottom Line or Public Health: Tactics Corporations Use to Influence Health and Health Policy, and What We Can Do to Counter Them.* London, UK: Oxford University Press.

World Health Organization (WHO). 2004. "Global Strategy on Diet, Physical Activity and Health." http://www.who.int/dietphysical activity/strategy/eb11344/en/index.html (accessed May 1, 2012).

World Health Organization (WHO). 2008. *2008-2013 Action Plan for the Global Strategy for the Prevention and Control of Non-Communicable Diseases: Prevent and Control Cardiovascular Diseases, Cancers, Chronic Respiratory Diseases and Diabetes.* Geneva, Switzerland: WHO Press.

World Health Organization (WHO). 2011. "Obesity and Overweight." http://www.who.int/mediacentre/factsheets/fs311/en/ (accessed March 26, 2012).

World Health Organization (WHO). 2012. "Health Impact Assessment (HIA)." http://www.who.int/hia/en/ (accessed May 1, 2012).

www.parliament.uk 2012a. "The Two-House System." http://www.parliament.uk/about/how/role/system/ (accessed March 30, 2012).

www.parliament.uk 2012b. "Members of Parliament." http://www.parliament.uk/about/mps-and-lords/members/ (accessed March 30, 2012).

Understanding the Role of Policy Narratives and the Public Policy Arena: Obesity as a Lesson in Public Policy Development

Randy S. Clemons, *Mercyhurst University*
Mark K. McBeth, *Idaho State University*
Elizabeth Kusko, *Idaho State University*

Introduction

As witnessed by recent national policy battles over healthcare and climate change, the policy environment in the United States is increasingly politically polarized. Whether this polarization occurs mainly among policy elites (e.g., Fiorina, Abram, and Pope 2010) or the mass public (e.g., Hunter 1992), U.S. public policy is progressively driven by divisive symbols (Miller and Fox 2007) and dominated by morality debates often articulated in the form of emotional narratives (Lakoff 2002). As the topic of obesity as a public health issue gained traction in the United States, we began to question how that issue would play out in the contemporary policy environment. Recently, increased attention has been given to the problem of obesity in the United States and its impact on the health and healthcare costs of the country. Indeed, this issue has been no stranger to morality debates and emotional diatribes.

First Lady Michelle Obama has been at the forefront of those treating obesity as a public policy issue. As the battle over healthcare raged on, her focus gradually shifted toward obesity and finally was formalized into her "Let's Move" campaign which targets childhood obesity (http://www.letsmove.gov/). Let's Move celebrated its second anniversary in February 2012. This campaign has undoubtedly witnessed success as by the passage of a fairly important piece of legislation (The Healthy, Hunger-free Kids Act of 2010) that promises progress toward reducing childhood obesity. In addition, obesity policy has not just focused at the national level, as at the state and local level of government, there has been much discussion in the last year of the need for more exercise programs, soda taxes, and banning certain foods. In the latter case, San Francisco essentially legislated Happy Meals out of existence (Bernstein 2010). As policy scholars watching these events unfold, we wondered in the vein of Baumgartner and Jones (1993) about the likelihood for a significant change in the government's role relative to obesity and, as a result, policy innovation that would be more than incremental.

While one will hardly ever reach 100% agreement on whether or not obesity constitutes a significant U.S. health concern (e.g., Campos 2004; Center for Consumer Freedom 2007), most experts accept that the concern is real and the debate today primarily regards the role of government in our lives, not whether obesity is a problem. For example, in the former context, U.S. Senator Tom Coburn asked the then U.S. Supreme Court nominee Elena Kagan whether or not Congress could use the Interstate Commerce Clause to pass a law forcing people to eat fruits and vegetables (Sargent 2010). Meanwhile, relative to the latter issue, well-known statistics continue to roll in: within the last two decades, among the 50 states and the federal district, Washington DC had the smallest percentage increase in obesity at 26%, while the other Washington (state) saw an incredible increase of 186%. The army has had to reject one in four of potential recruits due to obesity (Newsmax Health 2010). In the European Union (EU), weight gains have resulted in 15% of adults being obese (Kelland 2010), but in the

43

United States more than 33% of adults are obese (Center for Disease Control and Prevention 2012; Miller 2010). Given this evidence, obesity appears to be a largely unaddressed national health crisis impacting healthcare costs, economic productivity, and arguably even national security.

On the face of it, obesity appears as an "objective problem" with both economic and social implications. Contributing to health problems, obesity can affect healthcare costs (Centers for Disease Control and Prevention 2011) and worker productivity (Lippincott Williams & Wilkins 2008). Furthermore, obesity clearly harms children whose life chances are negatively impacted by being overweight, required to deal with the prejudices of a society that seems to simultaneously promote over-eating and the importance of being thin. Finally, individuals including the First Lady (Allen 2010) and Secretary of Agriculture Tom Vilsack (Jalonick 2010) have suggested that our national security may be threatened as U.S. citizens become overly obese: as noted earlier 25% of Americans who attempt to join the military are deemed unfit for military service due to obesity.

While many studies have examined the role of such demographic factors as race (e.g., Chambliss, Finley, and Blair 2004), gender (e.g., Chambliss, Finley, and Blair 2004), age (Hilbert, Rief, and Braehler 2008), and other factors on individual obesity attitudes, the research question that is explored in this paper does not ask whether obesity is a legitimate health problem, and thus the province of public health and medical experts. Nor is our research question relevant to obesity's causes and potential cures or what or who is factually to "blame" when an individual is obese. Nor do we directly focus on the constitutional and philosophical debate about federalism and the proper role of government, which is the province of public law scholars. Rather, we contend that the question of whether or not obesity will eventually become a problem leading to policy change and policy innovation does not depend solely, or primarily, on facts such as the extent of obesity and its negative consequences. Instead, we argue that for obesity to become defined and accepted as a public problem and for ensuing policy change to occur, public opinion toward obesity and the public's causal attribution (Weiner, Perry, and Magnusson 1988) comprise the key factors. Importantly, public health experts can benefit from both knowledge of how the public views obesity and from greater understanding of how the public policy process in the United States works in general. Ultimately, we believe that public opinion toward obesity and the government's role is, like much of contemporary U.S. public policy, grounded not in objective facts but rather in the realm of foundational beliefs about morality and in the question of individual versus community responsibility.

In today's media-driven policy environment, the battle over public opinion and obesity takes place on Internet blogs, in the visual realm of YouTube clips, and in other more traditional media outlets such as television, newspapers, and magazines. In fact, increasingly it is recognized that in the United States, public policy formation is heavily influenced by the role of policy narratives (or stories) that are told by various political actors in efforts to shape public opinion, and the academic literature has taken note of the importance of these policy narratives (e.g., Jones 2010; Jones and McBeth 2010; Verweij, et al. 2006). As described by Stone (2002), these policy narratives define a problem, cast certain individuals as heroes, villains, or victims, and normally conclude with a moral of the story (a solution). Additionally, policy narratives are often grounded in an underlying morality (Lakoff 2002) and the work of both Stone and Lakoff led us to our research question.

Specifically, we ask whether attitudes about obesity policy are grounded in an individual's moral foundation, as captured by Lakoff's parenting typology and in one's view of individual rights and responsibilities. We suggest that together these factors determine which obesity narrative an individual will buy into—either a narrative in which characters are active perpetrators of their own demise or innocent victims of larger forces. In short, we argue that the definition of obesity and obesity policy is ultimately grounded in political ideology, value-conflict, and morality (Saguy and Riley 2005) and as such obesity may constitute not an objective problem with medical and scientific-based solutions but rather an intractable or wicked problem (Rittel and Webber 1973).

Views of obesity in the United States are grounded in differing views of morality, the responsibility of the individual, and the government's fundamental role in the lives of citizens. Importantly, obesity involves the inherently personal act of eating, something traditionally viewed as an individual choice with individual consequences. In sum, as research using attribution theory has shown (e.g., Puhl and Brownell 2003; Weiner, Perry, and Magnusson 1988) many people accept a policy narrative claiming that obesity is not a structural or societal problem, but rather an individual one.

Thus, the policy battle over obesity and public opinion is likely to be one where obesity policy advocates will construct a policy narrative demonstrating that eating is not just an individual choice. Rather, our eating habits are constructed by multi-million dollar advertising campaigns and other corporate efforts designed to socially construct, but make appear "natural," eating habits that include supersized fast food and high fructose corn syrup-based food and drink. To influence public opinion, advocates of government obesity policy must demonstrate the "social construction" of what we eat. Just as anti-smoking advocates needed to demonstrate how smoking was not just an individual choice (due to the effects of advertising, pro-smoking images in popular culture, and ultimately the addictive nature of nicotine), to be successful in obesity policy, advocates must move the policy narrative and thus the perceptions of the act of eating from the individual as an independent agent toward the individual as a victim of other forces. Furthermore, advocates must construct policy narratives that expand the issue in order to show that obesity impacts society at large, not just large individuals. Just as anti-smoking advocates needed to demonstrate the healthcare costs of individual tobacco use and how the individual choice of smoking impacts others (most notably through second-hand smoke), obesity policy advocates must demonstrate the widespread nature of the costs of obesity across many groups. Even then, as with anti-smoking policy, if successful, such efforts will lead to intense political conflict between major corporate interests who have material interests in the outcome and those philosophically opposed to this narrative, e.g., those who view obesity policy as encroaching on parental or individual rights.

Our approach to research and general theoretical orientation accepts that public policy formation in the United States is not always a rational process (e.g., Baumgartner and Jones 1993; Clemons and McBeth 2009; Layzer 2006; Kingdon 1997) and is instead predominantly a process grounded in politics, political ideology, and beliefs. Thus, problems that might well be legitimately based in science can be ignored by government for many years while, conversely, other problems with less legitimacy and scientific backing might quickly move onto the government's institutional and decision agenda. While there are many different explanations of why problems do not become public problems, as narrative analysts we are predominately interested in how discussions of public policy in the United States are grounded in individual moral responsibility, in the form of narratives and how these narratives might impact public opinion. In other words, as Deborah Stone (2002) eloquently established, problems that are viewed as the acts of independent agents are unlikely to garner public attention. Therefore, as long as obesity is perceived as a "moral failing" the public attention and sympathies necessary for government support will not exist. A key question remains: what type of narrative is most convincing and effective? For example, a rational, scientific, evidence-based story; a compelling, anecdotal, individual is to blame story; or a compelling, anecdotal, society is to blame story.

Of course, there have been some policy decisions that affect obesity and there are plans in place to further government's role in promoting healthy eating. For example, as mentioned earlier, on February 9, 2010, the First Lady of the United States, Michelle Obama, announced plans for an anti-childhood obesity program named "Let's Move" (http://www.letsmove.gov/). The campaign, among other things, calls for better food labeling, more nutritious school lunch programs, and more exercise for children. Despite former Arkansas governor Mike Huckabee's plea that calls to end obesity should not be politicized and the rather innocuous policies promoted by "Let's Move," the First Lady's campaign has led to a series of criticisms of the program; from views on the left and in the medical community that Obama's program could lead to eating disorders, to critics on the right arguing that this epitomizes the nanny state and encroaching socialism (Jalonick 2010). One example was Sarah Palin's statement that it is an over-reaching of government's role in individual personal lives and her widely cited "s'mores" jab at Michelle Obama as being supposedly opposed to anyone eating desserts (Martin 2010).

The research that follows explores the role of policy narratives in the public policy process; and in building the theory of the roles that morality, responsibility/attribution, control, and fate play in public policy formation; with a subsequent literature review leading to testable hypotheses. Finally, we detail our survey methodology, present our results, discuss the results in the context of the academic literature and future research directions, and ultimately answer our overarching research question which, simply stated, asks which is most convincing and persuasive to individuals—a scientific statement, a narrative grounded in individual responsibility and the Strict Father Metaphor, or a narrative grounded in society responsibility and the Nurturing Parent Metaphor?

Theoretical Development: Narratives, Victims, Parenting, and Fate versus Control

The literature shows that there are many ways to study policy change and obesity. First, to become a public problem an issue such as obesity requires a legal and politically acceptable solution (Rochefort and Cobb 1993). A second possible approach that explains how obesity could become a public problem is found in the concept of market failures, one of the first lessons taught to policy analysts (Weimer and Vining 2004). The central lesson is that the government only gets involved in policy issues when the market fails and regulation is necessary to deal with externalities and other potential negative consequences of market transactions. Third, building on the long tradition of Multiple Streams Theory (Kingdon 1997), recent literature has stressed the importance of focusing events in bringing problems such as obesity to large-scale public attention (Birkland 2004; Clark 2004). As Kingdon argues, problems can be brought to public attention through academic studies and statistical measures. Yet, focusing events are powerful and tend to bring immediate attention to a policy problem.

Our interest, however, rests in the role that policy narratives play in shaping public opinion. Policy narratives are powerful tools in today's public policy arena, a policy arena that is increasingly dominated by policy marketing and ideas (e.g., Jones and McBeth 2010) thus making policy narratives and their study even more important in understanding the cacophony of noise that often obscures contemporary policy making.

Recent research has explored the power of narratives and what attributes make narratives particularly powerful. For example, research using experimental design (e.g., Ricketts 2007) demonstrates that narratives, similar to focusing events, are more powerful than traditional, rational techniques of persuasion such as science and statistics. Likewise, other studies show how individuals are more influenced by narratives than they are by science (e.g., Golding, Krimsky, and Plough 1992; Rook 1987; Small, Loewenstein, and Slovic 2007). For example, among these studies that demonstrate the power of narratives, using the issue of radon gas, Golding, Krimsky, and Plough (1992, 33) found that narrative formats of communication may be better at holding a reader's attention than more technical formats. Similarly, Small, Loewenstein, and Slovic (2006) use experimental design to demonstrate that individuals are more likely to give charitable contributions to an identifiable victim than to a statistical abstraction (also see Slovic 2007). In short, these findings (Small, Loewenstein, and Slovic 2006; Slovic 2007) demonstrate that individuals have more empathy for identifiable, individual victims as illustrated in a narrative than they do for abstractions such as groups. Finally, an additional element that explains the power of narratives is that individuals are attracted to stories that connect to an individual's identity. As illustrated in consumer marketing, marketing researchers know well the power of narrative as they strategically construct narratives that tap into a consumer's self-concept (e.g., Escalas 2004). This may well be important in public policy where research has shown that an individual's policy preferences are strongly tied to their cultural beliefs which in turn lead to what sources of information they trust or do not trust (Kahan, Jenkins-Smith, and Braman 2011).

The empirical evidence of the power of narratives versus scientific/statistical treatments is also mixed depending on the experimental design, the subject matter, the delivery method of the narrative, the type of narrative, and how outcomes are measured (self-reported behavior versus actual behavior, short-term knowledge versus long-term knowledge). Greene and Brinn (2003), for example, found that statistical messages about skin cancer outperformed narratives when it came to influencing a person's self-reported behavior and providing information. Marty and McDermott (1986) likewise found that a statistical treatment outperformed a narrative delivered personally when it came to increasing an individual's knowledge of testicular cancer. Ricketts (2007, 23-35) provides an excellent review of the conflicting studies on the power of narratives versus scientific and statistical statements.

However, we believe that the general findings regarding power of narratives contain implications for understanding why some public policy problems are ignored while other problems are addressed. This relates to the character of their narrative portrayals. In many ways, the findings reinforce the literature on the power of focusing events (e.g., Birkland 2004) in that individuals tend to ignore abstract warnings about "terrorism" or issues such as the health threat caused by fine particulate matter. Instead, individual views are more greatly impacted by events like September 11, 2001 with dramatic narratives involving identifiably innocent victims clearly not responsible for the tragic fate that befalls them. In public policy terms, narratives contribute to what Baumgartner and Jones (1993) refer to as a policy's image. A dominant narrative of an issue captures the issue's meaning and reduces complexity. Moreover, as policy narratives are composed of characters, plots, a structure, and a context (Jones and McBeth 2010; Stone 2002), they are utilized by policy entrepreneurs and others in a variety of policy tasks including design and implementation. Thus, the importance of narratives is magnified in a policy world increasingly dominated by marketing and symbolism (e.g., Miller and Fox 2007; Miller 2002). Policy narratives are composed of characters and plots, and a structure and a context (Jones and McBeth 2010; Stone 2002). Notably, the use of narratives in problem definition has long been insightfully discussed in the literature (Stone 2002).

While policy narratives are traditionally studied in post-structural terms (e.g., Fischer and Forrester 1993), increasingly narratives are a source of empirical policy study (e.g., McBeth, et al. 2007). Jones and McBeth (2010) introduce what they term a "Narrative Policy Framework" as an empirically driven hypothesis framework interested in causal theory at the micro and meso levels of analysis. Jones and McBeth (2010, 24) argue that "narratives must be anchored in generalizable content to limit variability." Furthermore, included in McBeth and Jones's list of belief systems that can be used to ground and test policy narratives is Lakoff's (2002) theory of parenting metaphors and morality. Lakoff's theory of moral politics contends that political ideology is strongly correlated with an individual's view of parenting. Conservatives rely on a "Strict Father Morality" (SFM) of parenting where the father is the absolute moral authority and where strict rules are used to teach individual responsibility (Lakoff 2002). Conversely, liberals rely on a "Nurturing Parent Morality" (NPM) that stresses mutual love, respect, and concern for others. Empirical research (Barker and Tinnick 2006) has shown some support for Lakoff's theory of predicting ideological predispositions of individuals.

Such a grounding in morality and parenting seems obviously important in a study of obesity, as morality and parenting likely play into an individual's view of obesity. Using the SFM, individuals might tend to see obesity as the result of lack of individual virtues such as self-control. Subsequently, this view of parenting would likely argue that the only solution to obesity is found not in public policy but rather in parents teaching individuals appropriate virtues. Conversely, supporters of the NPM would likely suggest that the causes of obesity are found more in social and environmental factors and that instead of blaming victims for their obesity, society and government policy should work to remove various conditions in the community (e.g., advertising and fast food) that contribute to and arguably cause individual obesity.

The research on parenting metaphors closely parallels work by Stone (2002) and Ingram, Schneider, and deLeon (2007) and, importantly, "attribution theory" (e.g., Rush 1998; Weiner, Perry, and Magnusson 1988). This latter psychology research is foundational in understanding how individuals either experience anger if they believe that a person wants help for a controllable condition, or conversely, how individuals will express pity and a desire to help those whose condition is outside of their control (Schmidt and Weiner 1988). Similarly, the central battle over the theory of causation in public policy is the question of fate versus control (Stone 2002). Essentially, innocent victims (fate) are seen as more "deserving and entitled" (Ingram, Schneider, and deLeon 2007) and are more likely to receive policy attention than "undeserving" individuals who play an active role in their own demise or problem (control). As such, the central role of a policy narrative in problem definition is this attribution of causation and delineating who is harmed by a specific problem and who is to blame. If individuals are shown to be "innocent" in their relation to a problem, the problem is more likely to receive public attention and support. Conversely, if an individual is an active participant in a problem, the problem is less likely to receive public attention and support. This suggests that there is a moral dimension of perceived responsibility versus victimization that often influences public opinion on an issue.

48

Examples of the moral dimension in public policy and the relationship of this morality to innocent or deserving victims are plentiful. For example, cigarette smoking was not historically viewed by the public as a problem requiring policy solutions, at least partially because smokers were viewed as individually responsible for individual consequences of cigarette smoking. This only changed when scientific studies demonstrated that second-hand smoke caused illness (and thus created innocent victims) and when studies showed that cigarette smokers were innocent victims of intentional tobacco company actions involving nicotine which tobacco companies apparently knew was addictive (see generally, Derthick 2001). Only then did the public acknowledge implications of the problem of cigarette smoking.

Another example of the moral dimension involved AIDS policy in the United States where heterosexual victims of blood transfusions (such as Ryan White and celebrities such as Arthur Ashe and Elizabeth Glaser) changed the problem definition of this deadly disease. As the definition changed so did public support for AIDS funding because blood transfusion recipients were viewed as innocent victims. This shift contrasted starkly to the U.S. AIDS policy narrative in the early 1980s that portrayed AIDS as a "Gay disease" with all the moral dimensions that go with such a definition (see generally, Shilts 1987). In addition and related to the last example, in a review of 32 years of survey findings, Lewis (2009) found that individuals are more tolerant of homosexuality when they believe that homosexuality has a biological basis rather than being a choice or preference. The idea is that individuals are more tolerant of homosexuality when people who are gay are in essence "innocent victims" of their own biology.

Thus, in today's obesity policy discussions, we would expect individuals to support public policy addressing obesity if they believed that obesity is outside of human control and instead is caused by genetics or environmental factors. We would further expect that individuals who subscribe to the NPM would be more likely to have such a view of obesity. Conversely, if individuals believe that obesity is the result of individual laziness or lack of self-control, we would expect that they subscribe to the SFM. Thus, obesity policy may come down to ideological differences, with conservatives opposing obesity policy and liberals supporting it. Such a dichotomy might be somewhat overdrawn, however. Recent research by Barry et al. (2009) finds that when given a choice, individuals will spread blame over several obesity metaphors. These metaphors range from "sinful behavior" (high blame) to "toxic food environment" (low blame) and individuals tend to spread blame across a range of individual responsibility to collective responsibility metaphors. Similarly, Brownell et al. (2010) argue that effective obesity policy must acknowledge and bridge both personal and collective responsibility while avoiding advocacy that focuses only on social responsibility.

Methodology

A survey (available upon request) was administered to students in social science courses at two separate schools of higher education. One school is public and located in the rural west United States; the second school is private and located in the northeast United States. The two schools are 1,900 miles apart. The Institutional Review Board at each school reviewed and approved the survey research. The survey consisted of questions measuring a respondent's parenting views (Barker and Tinnick 2006), political ideology, and other demographic variables. In addition, respondents answered questions about healthcare policy (taken from Oliver and Lee 2005). Each survey began with a separate description (two narratives and one statement) of the obesity issue. Our goal was not to test the impact of a narrative on attitudes in a classic pre-test/post-test experimental design. On the contrary, we were interested in how respondents rated the convincing nature of the narratives and the scientific statement, their morality (as measured in a Lakoff parenting scale), and their views on various statements about obesity policy. The methodology followed recent work by McBeth, Lybecker, and Garner (2010) and utilized a within-subjects design.

We presented two narratives and a scientific statement about obesity (see Appendix A). Our narrative choice is dichotomous because Lakoff presents his parenting metaphor as dichotomous and because we wanted a "forced choice" response option that asked each respondent to choose between either one of the narratives or the scientific statement. Such a methodological approach has advantages in that a forced choice might elicit more thought on behalf of the respondent who must choose what narrative or statement is most persuasive (Smyth et al. 2006). It also would be possible to create a "mixed" narrative that includes elements of both of Lakoff's metaphors and, in addition, some statistical evidence. For our purposes though, we wanted to find out if Lakoff's two distinctive metaphors could be turned into two distinctive narratives; again, Lakoff's discussion of these metaphors presents them as dichotomous. The SFM (see Appendix A) policy narrative presents some statistical evidence but is mainly focused on the character of "Kim" who does not exercise and overeats, and is thus presented in a way that largely sets up Kim to be perceived either as a villain or as an unsympathetic victim. In the SFM policy narrative, the moral of the story is that citizens like Kim must be taught at home to eat correctly and practice self-control. Ultimately, following Lakoff's lead, the solution is cast in terms of moral responsibility of the individual as the narrative directly rejects government policies to end obesity because such policies shift blame from the individual to society.

The NPM policy narrative (Appendix A), conversely, includes the same statistical evidence as the SFM narrative but presents the character Kim as an innocent victim and casts society as the villain. The narrative also defines the problem in terms of morality, but unlike the individual morality of SFM, this narrative presents an NPM societal morality. In this narrative, Kim can only afford to eat fast food and because of a demanding work schedule does not have the time to exercise. The narrative then asserts community responsibility for creating a healthy environment and proceeds to blame advertising for Kim's obesity. Finally, the narrative promotes several governmental solutions including regulating ads, taxing unhealthy foods, and removing unhealthy concessions from schools.

The science statement (Appendix A) simply lists statistics relating to obesity and the health consequences involved and then uses this evidence to declare that public health experts support taxing unhealthy food, regulating advertising, and removing unhealthy concessions from schools.

The two narratives and scientific statement were randomized to test for and avoid an ordering effect. After reading the description in the form of a story or scientific evidence, the respondents rated their agreement with various obesity statements. Below is a description of the survey in terms of dependent and independent variables.

Dependent Variables

1. Respondents were asked to choose the problem definition they found most convincing (choosing between the Strict Father narrative, Nurturing Parent narrative, and

science statement). Again, the choices were randomized to avoid and test for an order effect.

2. Rating (on a zero to six scale): obesity as a serious problem, regulating junk food ads, imposing snack taxes, eliminating fast food concessions from public schools, government takes too much care of people, individuals are responsible for what they eat, society contributes to obesity through advertising, the government has a role to play in reducing obesity.

Independent Variables

3. Morality Parenting index (serves as both a dependent and independent variable): summation of choices for: which is more important in children (independence or respect, curiosity or good manners, being considerate or being well-behaved). Respondents scored a zero for each Nurturing Parent response and a one for each Strict Father response. Thus, the index ranged from zero (strong Nurturing Parent) to three (strong Strict Father).

Control Variables

4. Partisan affiliation (scored on a seven point scale).
5. Ideological orientation (scored on a seven point scale).
6. Gender.
7. Age (measured in years).

Statistical Analysis

Our statistical treatment included descriptive statistics, chi-square, a *t*-test, correlation, and multiple regression (standardized coefficients with standard error reported).

Again, our interest is in the power of narratives, the usefulness of the parenting metaphor as a surrogate for political ideology, and whether there are distinctive Strict Father and Nurturing Parent narratives. We test four hypotheses:

H1: The two obesity narratives will be more persuasive to respondents than the science statement.

H2: There will be a relationship between a person's political ideology and their parenting metaphor.

H3: There will be an association between a person's parenting typology and choice of most persuasive obesity story or statement.

H4: There will be a relationship between support for various story elements and a person's parenting type.

Results

One hundred and seventy-two individuals completed the survey. This included 97 respondents from the northeastern, private, urban school and 75 from the western, public, rural school. Interestingly, there were no significant differences between the two samples in terms of their survey responses including their responses to demographic questions such as political ideology and partisanship. Overall, the sample was young and predominantly female but with varied political backgrounds. We did not ask a question about race but the sample was predominantly Caucasian. (See Appendix B for a more detailed background of respondents.)

Hypothesis #1: Stories are More Persuasive than Science

In Table 1, we find that 54% of respondents found the Strict Father story most convincing compared to only 21% who found the Nurturing Parent story most convincing. Twenty-five percent of respondents chose the science statement as most convincing. Thus, the scientific statement was slightly more convincing to respondents than the Nurturing Parent. Support for Hypothesis #1 is mixed.

Table 1 Choice of Most Persuasive Problem Definition

Story or statement	Frequency	Percent
Strict Father story	90	54.2
Nurturing Parent story	34	20.5
Science statement	42	25.3

Hypothesis #2: Relationship Between Parenting Metaphor and Political Ideology

In Table 2 we see descriptive data on the morality parenting index and data that demonstrates that there is a correlation between a person's score on the morality parenting index and political ideology (−0.190). Overall, 71 (43.5%) of the respondents were classified as following a nurturing parent morality and 92 (56.5%) were classified as following a strict father morality. As we had expected, the more conservative a respondent, the higher they scored (higher strict father) on the morality parenting index.

Table 2: The Parenting Index and Correlations with Political Ideology, Partisanship, Gender, and Age

Parenting metaphor	Frequency	Percent		
Strong nurturing	23	14.1		
Nurturing	48	29.4		
Strict father	64	39.3		
Strong strict father	28	17.2		
		Correlations		
	Ideology	Parenting	Gender	Age
Ideology	1	−0.190*	−0.027	0.111
Parenting	−0.190*	1	0.074	0.060
Gender	−0.027	0.074	1	−0.042
Age	0.111	0.060	−0.042	1

Note. *$p<0.05$.

Hypothesis #3: Association Between a Person's Parenting Typology and Choice of Most Persuasive Obesity Story or Statement

In Table 3 we find that 58.2% of the respondents categorized as preferring the "Strict Father" parenting approach chose the Strict Father story as most convincing to respondents compared with 48.5% of respondents categorized as preferring the Nurturing Parent approach who were most persuaded by the Strict Father story. Thirty-two percent of those categorized as Nurturing Parents chose the science statement as most convincing compared with only 22% of those categorized as a Strict Father. Nonetheless, the plurality of those identifying as nurturing parents chose the Strict Father Story. The calculated chi-square (2.091, df=2) was insignificant. We find no support for Hypothesis #3.

Table 3 Most Convincing by Parenting

Metaphor	SFM story	Nurturing story	Science statement
NPM	32 (48.5%)	13 (19.7%)	21 (31.8%)
SFM	53 (58.2%)	18 (19.8%)	20 (22%)
Total	85 (54%)	31 (19.7%)	41 (26.1%)
Chi-square (obtained)			
2.091, df=2			

Hypothesis #4: Relationship Between Support for Various Story Elements and a Person's Parenting Type

Table 4 presents the descriptive responses to the obesity statements. The statement "obesity is a serious problem" received strong support with a mean score of 5.50 (the scale ranged from 0, strongly disagree to 6, strongly agree, again see Appendix A). At the same time, the statement "individuals are responsible for what they eat or don't eat" also received strong support with a mean of 5.45.

The mean scores for the other statements were much more moderate and the standard deviations were much higher. The statement "society contributes to obesity advertising junk food" found moderate support with a mean score of 3.98. Likewise, the statement "there is too much advertising for junk food… and …the federal government should regulate these ads…" produced a mean of 3.58 with efforts to "eliminate fast food concessions" (3.58), producing a similar level of support. Respondents also had only some support for "government has a role to play in reducing obesity" (3.48). The statement that "government takes too much care of the people" also produced a mean of 3.30. Respondents did not support the "government snack tax" (2.79).

Table 4 Descriptive Statistics

Obesity statement	Mean	SD	n
Obesity is a serious problem	5.50	0.79	170
Regulate ads	3.91	1.67	170
Eliminate fast food concessions	3.58	1.72	170
Policies take care of people too much	3.30	1.59	169
Government-snack taxes	2.79	1.89	169
Individual responsibility	5.45	0.83	170
Society, junk food ads	3.98	1.38	169
Government has a role to play	3.48	1.44	170

In Table 5, the standardized coefficients produced in a multiple regression equation are presented. Here, surprisingly, the parenting morality index proves to be significantly related only to support of eliminating fast food concessions in public schools (−0.218) with Nurturing Parents more supportive of this measure. Political ideology (−0.349) was significantly related to the statement "government takes too much care of people" and "government has a role to play in obesity policy" (0.222) but surprisingly played no significant role in the other statements. Instead of the parenting metaphor and political ideology playing the predicted significant independent variable roles, gender (variable, Female) plays the most significant role with significant relationships to regulating ads (−0.186), eliminating fast food concessions (−0.231), imposing snack taxes (−0.230), society's role via advertising (−0.209), and government having a role to play in reducing obesity (−0.224). With each of these variables, females were more supportive than males. Thus, we find very limited support (nurturing parents support eliminating fast food concessions in public schools) for Hypothesis #4, which asserted that the parenting index would be related to a person's support of various obesity-related policy statements.

Table 5 Multiple Regression

	Parenting	Standardized coefficients (SE) Age	Female	Ideology
Serious problem	−0.141 (0.082)	0.061 (0.017)	−0.083 (0.150)	−0.037 (0.046)
Regulate ads	0.080 (0.155)	0.089 (0.033)	−0.186* (0.234)	0.161 (0.087)
Eliminate Concessions	−0.218** (0.164)	−0.003 (0.035)	−0.231** (0.301)	0.056 (0.092)
Policies take too much care	0.117 (0.115)	−0.033 (0.032)	0.154 (0.276)	−0.349** (0.085)
Snack taxes	−0.010 (0.181)	−0.046 (0.036)	−0.230** (0.332)	0.098 (0.102)
Individual responsibility	−0.043 (0.080)	−0.178* (0.017)	0.021 (0.147)	−0.118 (0.045)
Society and advertising	−0.044 (0.129)	0.080 (0.027)	−0.209* (0.237)	0.051 (0.072)
Government has role	−0.089 (0.131)	0.002 (0.028)	−0.224* (0.241)	0.222** (0.074)

Note. * $p \leq 0.05$; **$p \geq 0.01$.

Instead, we find that gender is the most important independent variable. Surprisingly, however, gender was not correlated with the morality parenting index. The data in Table 6 presents female and male scores for the seriousness of the obesity problem as well as for the various government policy options. Compared to males, females were more supportive of regulating ads, more supportive of snack taxes, more supportive of eliminating fast food concessions, and more in agreement that advertising contributes to obesity and that government has a role to play.

Table 6 Gender and Respondents' Views of Obesity

	Serious Mean SD *n*			Ads regulated Mean SD *n*			Taxes Mean SD *n*			Eliminate Mean SD *n*		
Female	5.56	0.81	99	4.17	1.4	99	3.10	1.9	98	3.90	1.6	99
Male	5.42	0.77	66	3.52	1.9	66	2.27	1.8	66	3.06	1.9	66
T-test	1.11			2.53*			2.81**			3.06**		
df	163			163			163			163		

	Take care	Responsible	Ad junk food	Gov. role
Female	3.20	5.46	4.22	3.64
Male	3.48	5.42	3.55	3.18
T-test	1.11	0.30	3.06**	2.03*
df	162	163	162	163

Note. **$p<0.01$; *$p<0.05$.

Key: Serious = Obesity is a serious problem, Ads regulated = ads should be regulated, Taxes = government imposed snack tax, Eliminate = eliminate fast-food and soft-drink concessions from schools, Takecare = government policies take too much care of people, Responsible = individuals are responsible for what they eat, Ad junk food = society contributes to obesity through advertising junk food, Gov role = government has a role to play.

Discussion

This initial study on the issue of obesity and the role of policy narratives produced both expected and unexpected results. First, consistent with our overall research orientation, the tenet comprised within Hypothesis #1, and literature (Golding, Krimsky, and Plough 1992; Ricketts 2007; Rook 1987; Small, Loewenstein, and Slovic 2006) that asserts the power of narratives, the Strict Father story was more convincing to respondents than was the scientific statement, though the scientific statement was more convincing than the Nurturing Parent story. Specifically, our first hypothesis posited that each of the obesity policy narratives (Strict Father or Nurturing Parent) would be more persuasive than the third option of a scientific statement. Our hypothesis is partially substantiated. Moreover, as Ricketts (2007) found narratives to be a more powerful tool of persuasion over the oft-thought arsenal of traditional techniques of rational science or statistics, we report some similar findings in support of the strength of policy narratives. Such a finding is surely unsettling for scientists, medical doctors, researchers, and others who are involved in health issues such as obesity. Yet, we also found that the content of the narrative itself matters. That is, the scientific statement was more persuasive than the Nurturing Parent narrative. Thus, our findings cannot be used to universally argue that narratives are more powerful than science. Instead, our limited data finds that some narratives are more powerful than science and science, in turn, is more powerful than some narratives. This, in general, is consistent with the divergent findings in the literature.

Second, consistent with the finding of Barker and Tinnick (2006) which demonstrates empirical support for Lakoff's theory of moral politics, political ideology, and the parenting metaphor, we find a correlation between the political ideology of a respondent and that respondent's parenting metaphor choice. Specifically, the more conservative the respondent's political ideology, the more likely they were to choose the Strict Father parenting morality metaphor. Contrastingly, the more liberal the respondent's political ideology the more likely they were to choose the Nurturing Parent morality metaphor. Essentially, such a finding provides further empirical evidence of Lakoff's parenting metaphor theory and its relationship to political ideology and moral/political decision making. Yet, more work needs to be done. Particularly, the three-item index borrowed from Barker and Tinnick (2006) appears limited.

Third, in regard to Hypothesis #4, which contends a relationship between support for various narrative or story elements and a respondent's parent metaphor choice, the Strict Father (conservative) narrative emphasizing individual responsibility over community responsibility was significantly more convincing to respondents than was either the Nurturing Parent narrative or the scientific statement. While the respondents agreed overall that obesity is a serious problem (mean score 5.50), the respondents believed that eating was a matter of individual responsibility rather than an appropriate realm for relevant governmental policy.

The latter finding (although limited to a sample of college students) provides some evidence that public opinion polls and, correspondingly, governmental policies might not deviate much from the status quo due to lack of a perceived "innocent victim." Among other factors, such as having a socially acceptable solution (Rochefort and Cobb 1993), strong evidence of market failure leading to the clear need for government regulation (Weimer and Vining 2004), and an event that focuses public attention (Birkland 2004), issues are more likely to be defined as a public problem when there are public perceptions that the issue's dominant story produces innocent victims (Stone 2002). Based on the findings from our limited sample, the issue of obesity appears to lack the innocent victim requirement and government's role, at least for now, is likely to remain limited to modifications of existing education programs impacting children and some health policies. Yet, there are other possibilities. A more nuanced narrative that incorporates both collective and individual responsibility (Brownell et al. 2010), as well as science, might well generate enough support to lead to meaningful policy change. Therefore, empirical research into the power of a more nuanced narrative would be a fruitful line for future inquiry.

Finally, multiple regression analysis finds that rather than a parenting preference or political ideology exerting independent variable significance, the factor of gender plays the most significant role in determining a person's support for government policies toward obesity.[1] Statistically, females are consistently more supportive of governmental policies, though both men and women found the seriousness of the problem equal and both comparably believed in individual responsibility. Thus, this study is consistent with other studies of obesity showing that gender influences attitudes toward obesity (e.g., Chambliss, Finley, and Blair 2004; Harris, Walters, and Waschull 1991).

Overall, developing an effective obesity policy narrative is a difficult challenge for public health policy advocates. First, there is the issue of defining obesity (Who are you calling fat?) that many citizens will defensively resist. Second, if obesity itself is defined as a problem, rather than high blood pressure, diabetes, or high cholesterol not only will a large number of citizens feel that they are under attack regardless of their individual healthiness, but also very different policy prescriptions will arise. Indeed, if obesity is as

---

[1] A preliminary statewide poll in Pennsylvania (USA) conducted by Mercyhurst University demonstrated ideological and partisan differences in regard to obesity policy but not gender.

widespread in the United States as the numbers suggest, telling any narrative about obesity is risky because it asks people to define their lifestyles and habits as harmful not only to themselves, but also to their children and to the common good. Thus, identifying obese children as innocent victims might motivate some people, but also could be seen as labeling their parents as villains. Third, the audiences' predispositions, in terms of foundational beliefs about morality, attribution, and about responsibility, may limit selling a narrative that leads to any dramatic change in public policy toward obesity.

Conclusion and Policy Implications

In conclusion, we return to our research question of "what is most convincing and persuasive to individuals—a scientific statement, a narrative grounded in individual responsibility, and the Strict Father Metaphor, or a narrative grounded in society responsibility and the Nurturing Parent Metaphor?" We posit the following answers based on our research.

Our initial evidence suggests that science plays only a limited role in convincing individuals that obesity is a policy problem. Instead, we found that a policy narrative based on individual moral responsibility was more convincing to individuals than was a scientific statement. Again, such findings might prove unsettling for those charged with addressing obesity as a medical issue worthy of public and government attention. Thus, even among liberal, nurturing parent respondents, views of obesity were most shaped by a story that holds the individual as morally and individually responsible for their lifestyle choices (e.g., poor diet and lack of exercise). Obesity policy advocates, as our limited data suggests, have also failed to demonstrate that solutions to obesity are socially acceptable.

We can also expect that advocates of obesity policy will attempt to reconstruct the narrative of obesity in the direction of the obese as an innocent victim of not only society but also genetics and other factors; and thus, as an innocent victim, be worthy of government intervention. Furthermore, obesity advocates will attempt to expand the issue of obesity by demonstrating widespread costs that go beyond the individual to larger societal costs affecting many more individuals, groups, and society as a whole. All of this provides ample research opportunities and future direction for students of public policy, particularly those interested in the political battles, policy narratives, and underlying morality stories that surround such issues.

Appendix A: Obesity Narratives and Scientific Statement

Scientific Statement

A recent study has revealed that one in five U.S. teenagers have cholesterol problems. In addition, a few years ago, the U.S. Surgeon General stated in 2003 that two out of every three Americans are overweight and illnesses related to obesity cost society more the longer people live. The health consequences of obesity are many including heart disease, cancer, Type II diabetes, and many other life-threatening illnesses. Public health experts have declared that America's over-eating is an epidemic and have suggested several policies including regulating advertising of food, taxing unhealthy foods, and removing unhealthy concessions from schools.

Strict Father Narrative

Historically, in the United States, our society has emphasized individual responsibility, hard work, and self-discipline. Yet, a recent study has revealed that one in five U.S. teenagers have cholesterol problems and the U.S. Surgeon General a few years earlier stated that two out of every three Americans are overweight and illnesses related to obesity cost society more the longer people live. Obesity in the United States is the result of a breakdown of individual responsibility, hard work, and discipline. For example, Kim Anderson is 20 years old and at 5 foot 11 inches tall, Kim weighs over 320 pounds with a total cholesterol level of over 300 (where 200 pounds is considered normal). He eats fast food every day, never exercises, and even drives his car to work even though he only lives three blocks from his place of employment. Kim Anderson, like other citizens, must be taught at home to eat correctly, exercise, and practice self-control over their eating habits rather than actively participating in destructive behavior. Citizens must take moral responsibility for their over-eating. Government policies such as banning advertising, taxing unhealthy foods, and removing unhealthy concessions from schools only contributes to the problem by shifting blame from individuals to society. It is up to individuals to improve their eating habits and health and government should not play a role.

Nurturing Parent Narrative

Society has tremendous responsibilities toward its children. For instance, a recent study has revealed that one in five U.S. teenagers have cholesterol problems and the U.S. Surgeon General stated a few years earlier that two out of every three Americans are overweight and illnesses related to obesity cost society more the longer people live. Obesity in the United States is the result of our society's lack of moral commitment to creating healthy environments for its citizens. For example, Kim Anderson is 20 years old and at 5 foot 11 inches tall, Kim weighs over 320 pounds with a cholesterol level of over 300 (where 200 pounds is considered normal). Because he works two low paying retail jobs, Kim can only afford to eat unhealthy cheap fast food and because of his work schedule he cannot find time to exercise. Citizens, like Kim, should be able to live in a larger community that encourages healthy eating instead of being manipulated by advertising. Businesses should not be allowed to dictate what citizens eat through their advertising and promotion of unhealthy eating choices. Government policies such as regulating advertising, taxing unhealthy foods, and removing unhealthy concessions from schools leads to a healthier environment for citizens and will reduce obesity.

Appendix B Demographics and Political Characteristics of the Sample

School	n	%	Gender	n	%	Age*	n	%
Urban	97	56%	Female	99	59%	18–22	134	81%
Rural	75	44%	Male	67	41%	23–29	23	14%
						30–36	7	4%
						37+	2	1%

Partisanship	n	%	Political Ideology	n	%	Vote (2008)	n	%
Republican	57	44%	Conservative	50	35%	McCain	23	14%
Independent	30	23%	Moderate	40	28%	Obama	31	19%
Democratic	44	36%	Liberal	52	37%	Other	1	0%
						Did not	25	15%
						Could not	87	53%

Missing values: Female (6), Age (6), Partisanship (41), Ideology (30), and Vote (5). We calculated percentages based on those reporting in each category.

*Age was reported in years as an interval-ratio variable. It was put into categories for this appendix.

**Political ideology was assessed with a seven-point Likert scale and collapsed here for presentation purposes.

References

Allen, M. 2010. "Michelle Obama has New Warning on Obesity." *Politico.* http://www.politico.com/news/stories/1210/46303.html (accessed February 23, 2011).

Barker, D.C., and J.D. Tinnick III. 2006. "Competing Visions of Parental Roles and Ideological Constraint." *American Political Science Review* 100 (2): 249-263.

Barry, C.L., V.L. Brescoll, K.D. Brownell, and M. Schlesinger. 2009. Obesity Metaphors: How Beliefs about the Causes of Obesity Affect Support for Public Policy." *The Milbank Quarterly: A Multidisciplinary Journal of Population Health and Health Policy* 87 (1): 7-47

Baumgartner, F.R. and B.D. Jones. 1993. *Agendas and Instability in American Politics.* Chicago: University of Chicago Press.

Bernstein, S. 2010. "San Francisco Bans Happy Meals." http://articles.latimes.com/2010/nov/02/business/la-fi-happy-meals-20101103 (accessed February 23, 2011).

Birkland, T.A. 2004. "The World Changed Today: Agenda Setting and Policy Change in the Wake of the September 11 Terrorist Attacks." *Review of Policy Research* 21(2): 179-200.

Brownell, K.D., R. Kersh, D.S. Ludwig, R.C. Post, R.M. Puhl, M.B. Schwartz, and W.C. Willett. 2010. "Personal Responsibility and Obesity: A Constructive Approach to a Controversial Issue." *Health Affairs* 29 (3): 379-387.

Campos, P. 2004. *The Obesity Myth: Why America's Obsession with Weight is Hazardous to Your Health.* New York: Gotham.

Center for Disease Control and Prevention. 2011a. "U.S. Obesity Trends." http://www.cdc.gov/obesity/data/trends.html (accessed February 23, 2011).

Center for Disease Control and Prevention. 2011b. "Economic Consequences." http://www.cdc.gov/obesity/causes/economics.html (accessed February 23, 2011).

Center for Disease Control and Prevention. 2012. "U.S. Obesity Trends." http://www.cdc.gov/obesity/data/trends.HTML (accessed February 12, 2012).

Center for Consumer Freedom. 2007. *Small Choices, Big Bodies.* Washington, DC: Center for Consumer Freedom. http://www.obesitymyths.com/Downloads/SCBB.pdf (accessed February 1, 2011).

Chambliss, H.O., C.E. Finley, and S.N. Blair. 2004. "Attitudes Toward Obese Individuals Among Exercise Science Students." *Medicine & Science in Sports & Exercise* 36 (3): 468-474.

Clark, B.C. 2004. "Agenda Setting and Issue Dynamics: Dam Breaching on the Lower Snake River." *Society and Natural Resources* 17: 599-699.

Clemons, R.S. and M.K. McBeth. 2009. *Public Policy Praxis: A Case Approach for Understanding Policy and Analysis.* New York: Longman.

Derthick, M.A. 2001. *Up in Smoke: From Legislation to Litigation in Tobacco Politics.* Washington, DC: CQ Press.

Escalas, J.E. 2004. "Narrative Processing: Building Consumer Connections to Brands." *Journal of Consumer Psychology* 14 (1 and 2): 168-180.

Fiorina, M.P., Abrams, S.J., and Pope, J.C., 2010. *Culture War? The Myth of A Polarized America,* Third Edition. New York: Longman.

Fischer, F. and J. Forrester. 1993. *The Argumentative Turn in Policy Analysis*. Durham: Duke University Press.

Golding, D., S. Krimsky, and A. Plough. 1992. "Evaluating Risk Communication: Narrative vs. Technical Presentations of Information About Radon." *Risk Analysis* 12 (1): 27-35.

Greene, K. and L.S. Brinn. 2003. "Influencing College Women's Tanning Bed Use: Statistical Versus Narrative Evidence Format and a Self-Assessment to Increase Perceived Susceptibility. *Journal of Health Communication* 8: 443-461.

Harris, M.B., L.C. Walters, S. Waschull. 1991. "Gender and Ethnic Differences in Obesity-Related Behaviors and Attitudes." *Journal of Applied Social Psychology* 21 (19): 1545-1566.

Hilbert, A., W. Rief, and E. Braehler. 2008. "Stigmatizing Attitudes Toward Obesity in a Representative Population-based Sample" *Obesity* 16 (7): 1529-1534.

Hunter, J.D. 1992. *Culture Wars: The Struggle to Define America*, New York: Basic Books.

Ingram, H., A.L. Schneider, and P. deLeon. 2007. "Social Construction and Policy Design." In *Theories of the Policy Process*, Second Edition, ed. Paul A. Sabatier. Boulder, CO: Westview Press.

Jalonick, M.C. 2010. "Congress Sends Child Nutrition Bill to Obama." http://news.yahoo.com/s/ap/20101202/ap_on_bi_ge/us_congress_child_nutrition (accessed February 23, 2011).

Jones, M.D. 2010. Heroes and Villains: Cultural Narratives, Mass Opinions, and Climate Change. Dissertation, PhD, Political Science, University of Oklahoma.

Jones, M.D. and M.K. McBeth. 2010. "Narrative Policy Framework: Clear Enough to be Wrong?" *Policy Studies Journal* 38 (2): 329-353.

Kahan, D.M., H. Jenkins-Smith, and D. Braman. 2011. "Cultural Cognition of Scientific Consensus." *Journal of Risk Research* 14: 1-28.

Kelland, K. 2010. "Half of Europe's Adults Overweight or Obese: Report." http://www.reuters.com/article/idUSTRE6B62B020101207 (accessed February 23, 2011).

Kingdon, J.W. 1997. *Agendas, Alternatives, and Public Policies*, Second Edition. New York: Longman.

Lakoff, G. 2002. *Moral Politics: How Liberals and Conservatives Think,* Second Edition. Chicago: University of Chicago Press.

Layzer, J. 2006. "Fish Stories, Science, Advocacy, and Policy Change in New England Fishery Management." *Policy Studies Journal* 34 (1): 59-80.

Lewis, G.B. 2009. "Does Believing Homosexuality is Innate Increase Support for Gay Rights?" *Policy Studies Journal* 37 (4): 669-693.

Lippincott Williams & Wilkins. 2008. "Obesity Linked to Reduced Productivity at Work." *Medical News Today*. http://www.medicalnewstoday.com/releases/93402.php. (accessed February 10, 2011).

Martin, R.S. 2010. "Palin's Reckless Views on Obesity." http://www.cnn.com/2010/OPINION/11/24/martin.michelle.obama.palin/index.html?hpt =T2 (accessed February 23, 2011).

Marty, P.J. and R.J. McDermott. 1986. "Three Strategies for Encouraging Testicular Self-Examination among College Aged Males." *Health Education* 16: 33-36.

McBeth, M.K., D.L. Lybecker, K. Garner. 2010. "The Story of Good Citizenship: Framing Public Policy in the Context of Duty-Based versus Engaged Citizenship." *Politics & Policy* 38 (1): 1-23.

McBeth, M.K., E.A. Shanahan, R.J. Arnell, P.L. Hathaway. 2007. "The Intersection of Narrative Policy Analysis and Policy Change Theory." *Policy Studies Journal* 35 (1): 87-108.

Miller, H.T. 2002. *Postmodern Public Policy*. Albany: State University of New York Press.

Miller, H.T., and C.J. Fox. 2007. *Postmodern Public Administration*. New York: M. E. Sharpe.

Miller, L. 2010. "Divided We Eat." *Newsweek*, November 29: 42-48.

Newsmax Health. 2010. "Military: 1 in 4 Recruits Too Fat or Uneducated to Serve." http://www.newsmaxhealth.com/health_stories/Obesity_Military/2010/12/23/368277.html (accessed February 10, 2011).

Newsweek, 2010. "Who's the Fattest in the Land", December 20: 12.

Oliver, J.E. and Taeku Lee. 2005. "Public Opinion and the Politics of Obesity in America." *Journal of Public Health Politics, Policy and Law* 30 (5): 923-954.

Puhl, R.M. and K.D. Brownell. 2003. "Psycho-Social Origins of Obesity Stigma: Toward Changing a Powerful and Pervasive Stigma." *Obesity Reviews* 4: 213-227.

Ricketts, M.S. 2007. The Use of Narratives in Safety and Health Communication. Doctoral Dissertation. The University of Kansas, Department of Psychology

Rittel, H.W.J. and M.M. Webber. 1973. Dilemmas in a General Theory of Planning. *Policy Sciences* 4: 155-169.

Rochefort, D.A. and R.W. Cobb. 1993. "Problem Definition, Agenda Access and Policy Choice." *Policy Studies Journal* 21 (1): 56-71.

Rook, K.S. 1987. "Effects of Case History versus Abstract Information on Health and Behaviors." *Journal of Applied Social Psychology* 17: 533-553.

Rush, L.L. 1998. "Affective Reactions to Multiple Social Stigmas." *Journal of Social Psychology*, 138: 421-430.

Sargent, G. 2010. "Big Sis Elena Kagan Wants to Tell You What to Eat? *Washington Post*. http://voices.washingtonpost.com/plum-line/2010/06/gop_big_sis_elena_kagan_is_wat.html (accessed February 23, 2011).

Saguy, A.C. and K.W. Riley. 2005. "Weighing Both Sides: Mortality, Mortality and Framing Contests over Obesity." *Journal of Health Politics, Policy and Law* 30 (5): 869-921.

Schmidt, G. and B. Weiner. 1988. "An Attribution-Affect-Action Theory of Motivated Behavior: Replications of Judgments of Help-Giving." *Personality and Social Psychology Bulletin*, 14 (3): 610-621.

Shilts, R. 1987. *And the Band Played On: Politics, People and the AIDS Epidemic*. New York: St. Martin's Press.

Slovic, P. 2007. "If I Look at the Mass I will Never Act: Psychic Numbing and Genocide." *Judgment and Decision Making* 2 (2): 79-95.

Small, D.A., G. Loewenstein and P. Slovic. 2007. "Sympathy and Callousness: The Impact of Deliberative thought on Donations to Identifiable and Statistical Victims." *Organizational Behavior and Human Decision Processes* 102: 143-153.

Smyth, J.D., D.A. Dillman, L.M. Christian, and M.J. Stern. 2006. "Comparing Check-All and Forced-Choice Question Formats in Web Surveys." *Public Opinion Quarterly* 70 (1): 66-77.

Stone, D. 2002. *Policy Paradox: The Art of Political Decision Making*, Revised Edition, Third Edition. New York: W. W. Norton.

Verweij, M., M.D. Douglas, R. Ellis, C. Engel, F. Hendriks, S. Lohmann, S. Ney, S. Rayner, and M. Thompson. 2006. "Clumsy Solutions for a Complex World: The Case of Climate Change." *Public Administration* 84 (4): 817-843.

Weimer, D. and A.R. Vining. 2004. *Policy Analysis: Concepts and Practice*, Fourth Edition. New Jersey: Prentice Hall.

Weiner, B., R.P. Perry, and J. Magnusson. 1988. "An Attributional Analysis of Reactions to Stigma." *Journal of Personality and Social Psychology* 55 (5): 738-748.

II. Substance Control

Marijuana Legalization: Lessons from the 2012 State Proposals

Jonathan P. Caulkins, *Carnegie Mellon University*
Anna M. Kasunic, *Carnegie Mellon University*
Michael A. C. Lee, *Carnegie Mellon University*

Introduction

On November 6, 2012, citizens in three states will vote on whether to legalize production, distribution, and sale of marijuana for general—not just medical—use. Although federal prohibition would continue, this step would still be unprecedented; no developed polity in the modern era has legalized marijuana.[1] National polls presently show a nearly 50/50 split in public support for legalization (Newport 2011) with generally greater support in states with current legalization proposals.

There is ample literature on marijuana legalization in the abstract (e.g., Kleiman 1989; Caputo and Ostrum 1994; MacCoun and Reuter 2001; Rolles 2010; Room et al. 2010). This chapter complements such prior work by analyzing the specific proposals in play in 2012 and the possible consequences of state-level legalization in the face of ongoing federal prohibition. This analysis suggests that legalization in just one state could have a significant impact on price and use nationwide. Legalization in just one state might not be stable either; it could create conditions that would make other states more likely to follow. Thus, marijuana legalization is salient for all states, not just those considering changes this year.

This analysis examines how state-level marijuana legalization could affect marijuana use, which presumably translates into effects on use-related outcomes. It does not attempt to model the use-to-outcomes link itself. For example, we do not discuss how long-term marijuana use might influence cognitive functioning or lung health. This is analogous to trying to understand how a policy change might affect cigarette smoking prevalence without delving into how cigarettes affect health outcomes.

Synopsis of Standard Marijuana Legalization Analysis[2]

The marijuana legalization debate is often couched in terms of core values. For example, libertarians might argue that adults should be free to consume anything they like, even if that consumption is harmful. Various religions oppose such logic, condemning many intoxicants as intrinsically immoral.

However, legalization can also be considered on consequentialist grounds. Kleiman (1992) observes that the basic tradeoff is between amounts of use-related harms on the one hand, and amounts of black market-related harms on the other. Prohibition reduces availability and use. (Even marijuana—by far the most widely consumed illegal drug—is

---

[1] In the Netherlands, use, retail sale of up to 5 g, and personal cultivation are effectively legal. However, production, wholesale, and commercial processing remain entirely illegal.
[2] This section summarizes broad outlines of the standard analysis of marijuana legalization. We claim no original contribution, but seek merely to place the subsequent discussion in context.

used much less commonly than two legal drugs: tobacco and alcohol.) However, illegality cannot eliminate use, and the remaining illicit use tends to be riskier. Illegal markets also generate their own harms, including crime, violence, corruption, and the societal costs of efforts to suppress them.

A liberal[3] society generally presumes that adult consumers look after their own welfare, so government interference with the free market's invisible hand necessarily makes society worse off, absent market failures. For psychoactive drugs, externalities and dependence complicate that calculus.

Negative externalities are harms that use imposes on nonusers. Some substances generate harms primarily for the users; notwithstanding valid concerns about secondhand smoke, cigarette smokers themselves suffer most of the health consequences of tobacco. In contrast, drunk drivers kill and injure many innocent people. Marijuana use is generally seen to be more like tobacco in this regard; whatever the harms, they primarily affect users, not second or third parties.

Dependence raises the possibility of *internalities*. As defined in behavioral economics (Herrnstein et al. 1993), internalities are harms that users inflict on themselves without fully considering them before consumption. Standard economics overlooks this possibility with its devotion to consumer sovereignty, but internalities are a contributing motive behind many public health interventions.

The debate on marijuana's physical and mental health effects has lasted decades without consensus. The main concerns pertain to impaired driving, cancer, respiratory problems like emphysema, and mental health problems like schizophrenia. Insofar as consensus has been reached, it is that there are adverse health effects, but they are smaller than corresponding risks for other substances, notably alcohol.

The greater concern is *behavioral toxicity*. For example, marijuana use is correlated with greater school dropout rates and reduced labor productivity, raising concern that the association could be partially causal.

Behavioral toxicity includes risk of dependence. Relatively few people become dependent on marijuana. Indeed, 40–50% of those who have ever tried marijuana report fewer than 12 days of total lifetime use. Nevertheless, about 4.4 million people in the United States currently meet the clinical definition for marijuana abuse or dependence (roughly one-quarter of past-month users). The conventional view is that marijuana dependence is qualitatively different—and less debilitating—than dependence on some other substances (Room et al. 2010). However, hundreds of thousands of people seek marijuana treatment each year, and frequent users are exposed to a disproportionate share of the traditional forms of toxicity. Those who report using more than weekly in the last year account for 90% of all reported days of use,[4] and about half of them meet the criteria for abuse or dependence (Caulkins et al. 2012).

Some legalization advocates may disagree, but given the combined behavioral and physical toxicity of marijuana use, we believe a consumption increase would certainly merit public health concern.

---

[3] The classical term "liberal" means to favor markets largely free from government intervention.
[4] Days-of-use is a measure of quantity consumed. Survey respondents can answer with reasonable reliability how many days they used in the last week, month, or year, but have difficulty answering in terms of quantity (weight) consumed. Because of the skewed distribution of use—the minority of frequent users consume most of the drugs—it is important to use some measure of intensity of use, rather than looking only at past-year or past-month prevalence.

Crime is another prominent feature in legalization debates, but is much less central for marijuana since the United States has not experienced substantial violent crime around the illegal sale of marijuana. Like any intoxicant, marijuana can affect behavior, potentially leading users to take undue risks. But, unlike alcohol use, marijuana use is not associated with an increase in aggression according to several studies (e.g. White 1998). Likewise, while dependent heroin users may spend three-quarters of all of their income buying heroin (Roddy et al. 2011), marijuana purchases rarely dominate a user's budget, so its use is less associated with robbery and other income-generating crimes.

There is also the question of whether marijuana legalization could reduce the horrific drug violence in Mexico. The U.S. government had published an estimate that 60% of Mexican drug trafficking organizations' profits came from marijuana, but later retracted it. Kilmer et al. (2012) argue that the true portion is closer to 20%.

The scientific debate continues as to whether marijuana use has long-term cognitive effects, but some studies deem subtle effects at least probable (e.g., Hall 1994). Effects on youth matter because important cognitive areas guiding personality development, decision-making, and problem-solving are still maturing during adolescence (Thompson 2001). Psychoactive chemicals may harm the maturation process. It is worth noting also that younger marijuana users are more likely than those who delay initiation until adulthood to eventually become dependent.

Links with use and abuse of other drugs, including via the so-called gateway effect, are also prominent themes in legalization debates. Concern has ebbed somewhat about the classical version of the gateway theory, namely that youthful experimentation with marijuana *causes* increased risk of subsequent abuse of other drugs. Observational studies show that marijuana use almost universally predates harder drug use, but this phenomenon is now recognized as an association, not an indication of causality (e.g., Morral et al. 2002). Precocious marijuana use may be merely indicative of a person who is more disposed to partake in riskier behavior or engage in substance abuse (Caulkins et al. 2012).

Indeed, legalization advocates sometimes argue that legalizing marijuana will eliminate another "gateway" effect. Consumption of illegal marijuana necessitates interaction with and exposure to drug dealers who may also be willing and able to supply other drugs. If we legalize marijuana, so the argument goes, we eliminate that gateway effect.

Different frequencies of marijuana use during adolescence could carry various unique risks. The possibility of youthful *experimentation* with marijuana (indicated, say, by lifetime prevalence) causing subsequent problems is distinct from the possibility of adolescent marijuana *dependence* causing (not just being associated with) subsequent problems. This is less studied, but not unimportant. Household surveys estimate that the number of youth (under age 18) who meet clinical criteria for marijuana abuse or dependence (SAMHSA 2012) approaches one million, and it is generally believed that surveys underestimate problematic use. So if legalization caused an across-the-board increase in use, the number of additional youth who would meet these criteria for abuse or dependence could not be assumed to be small.

Interestingly though, most of the recent increase in U.S. marijuana consumption has been among adults. The total number of past-year use-days reported by adults has doubled, whereas under-18 use has barely budged. If these trends stem from liberalization (e.g., proliferation of medical dispensaries) and they continue after legalization, then perhaps legalization's larger effect could be delaying the average age at which recreational use ceases, rather than reducing the age of first use.

A final health outcome worth flagging is the effect legalization will have on alcohol abuse, since aggregate alcohol-related harms dwarf marijuana-related harms, according to current estimates (Harwood et al. 2000; ONDCP 2004). How marijuana legalization might alter alcohol-related social harms is as yet unknown. If marijuana substitutes for alcohol, then reductions in crime and other alcohol-related harms could prove to be marijuana legalization's greatest benefit. But if marijuana acts as a complement to alcohol, even modest increases in alcohol-related harms could more than offset any marijuana-related benefits of legalizing (Caulkins et al. 2012).[5] If consuming both together intensifies certain effects, the harms that those effects generate could become accentuated, and lead to an increase in their respective social costs. For example, several studies have found that tandem use of alcohol and marijuana exacerbates driving impairment (e.g., Robbe 1998), so greater tandem use would lead to more impaired driving accidents. (Despite decades of research on cross-price elasticities of demand and poly-drug abuse, it remains unclear whether marijuana is, on net, a substitute or a complement for alcohol or other drugs.)

Of late, fiscal outcomes have also figured prominently in the legalization debate because of the potential for increased tax revenue and decreased enforcement costs[6] (though both are often overstated). These outcomes are not a direct concern for public health, but they merit extended discussion because of the pivotal role they may play with regard to voter support and potential passage. Taxes matter also because they raise price, which can discourage use.

Legalization Proposals in the United States in 2012

Marijuana legalization is often conceived of as a binary choice, but that oversimplifies the issues. As of March 2012, 10 U.S. states were considering 17 proposals to legalize marijuana, including 14 voter initiatives and 3 legislative bills (in New Hampshire, Massachusetts, and Washington). These proposals are not at all alike; the details of each would have far different implications.

These proposals are in addition to the comparable number of proposals to create or extend medical marijuana regimes. They go well beyond decriminalization, which is typically defined as imposing civil rather than criminal penalties for possession of small amounts (Pacula et al. 2005). (Decriminalizing marijuana is not a radical step; more than a dozen U.S. states have already done it, some as early as the 1970s.[7]) These 17 proposals would legalize commercial cultivation, processing, distribution, sale, and possession of larger amounts—some just for those with licenses, others for all adults.

---

[5] Parallel reasoning could apply to tobacco and "hard" drugs.

[6] Harvard economist Jeff Miron (2010) estimated that enforcing marijuana prohibition costs the US$13.7B, with California's share being $1.87B. However, the estimate rests on a number of dubious assumptions, such as that marijuana-related prison costs can be computed by pro-rating total drug-related prison costs across drugs in proportion to the number of sales/manufacturing arrests by drug. Other estimates for California are an order of magnitude lower (Gieringer 2009a; 2009b at $204M; Caulkins and Kilmer, forthcoming at $150M for enforcing marijuana laws against those 21 and older). Miron (2012) himself subsequently observed that the magnitude of the cost savings is sometimes overstated by advocates, calling claims of a huge budgetary windfall problematic.

[7] Alaska, the most liberal state in terms of current marijuana laws, allows residents to possess up to 4 ounces and cultivate up to 25 plants for personal use.

This elementary fact is obvious when reading the proposals, but is nonetheless not widely appreciated. Even the venerable *New York Times* described Colorado's Regulate Marijuana like Alcohol Act as "a ballot proposal to *legalize possession of marijuana in small amounts* in Colorado..." [emphasis added] (Johnson January 26th, 2011). Again, on February 27th, the *Times* reported that "[a] voter initiative that *would legalize the possession of marijuana* by adults for recreational use qualified for [Colorado's] November ballot... Moves to *decriminalize* marijuana face opposition from the federal government..." [emphasis added] (Reuters 2011).

Those are fair characterizations of Section 3 of Colorado's proposition, which addresses personal use, but it is as if the reporters stopped reading at that point and were oblivious to Sections 4 (on "Lawful operation of marijuana-related facilities") and 5 (on regulation).

Political Viability

Passage of any one of the proposals is distinctly possible, but not equally likely; indeed, many have no realistic prospects of passing. As of this writing, three of the voter initiatives had gathered enough signatures to make the ballot: Colorado's Regulate Marijuana like Alcohol Act (henceforth shortened to "CO-RLA" for Colorado Regulate like Alcohol), Washington State Initiative 502 (WA I-502), and the Oregon Cannabis Tax Act (OCTA); they are the focus below.

Recent polls have support for legalization in Colorado hovering around 50%, with polls showing increasing support between June and August 2012 (Public Policy Polling). Support for legalization in Washington is also close to 50%, with the proportion of undecided voters as high as 7% (J. Martin 2012).

Oregon has already legalized medical marijuana, though in recent years proposals to provide for medical marijuana dispensaries have been voted down. Given the demographics and political leanings of Oregon's voters (according to Gallup, 26.4% liberal and 33.6% moderate in 2011), one might guess that OCTA has a reasonable chance of passing.

California is noteworthy for not having a proposal on the ballot even though its Proposition 19 dominated legalization discussions in 2010 (Kilmer et al. 2010a; 2010b). Proposition 19 gained 46.5% of the vote, with exit polls revealing that an additional 6% of voters chose to vote against it even though they favored marijuana legalization generally (Caulkins et al. 2012).

Supporters in California circulated several legalization initiatives for signatures, but were unable to coalesce around any one, and no initiative gathered the requisite 504,760 signatures by the March 26, 2012 deadline. California's Regulate Marijuana like Wine proposal (CA-RMLW) made the most progress towards that goal, so we include it in parts of the analysis below.

Propositions are an exercise in direct democracy. However, getting on the ballot depends on more than the intrinsic popularity of a measure. Attracting the attention of a few well-heeled donors can be critical, particularly in a large state. This year's events in California are telling in this regard. In a last-ditch effort to rally support behind a single initiative, advocates held a February summit that they dubbed "Cannadome," which carried an "all enter, one leaves" message. Proponents of the three most prominent proposals—Regulate Marijuana Like Wine, the Repeal Cannabis Penalties Act, and the Cannabis Hemp and Health Initiative—issued a statement of unity that said:

> We invite any freedom loving American with some serious assets to take a look at all three of our initiatives. Choose the one that you are willing to finance. The other two initiatives will support the one you choose 100% to ensure a victory in 2012. (M. Martin 2012)

The Cannadome appeal failed, but it highlights the disproportionate influence a few people with "serious assets" can have in determining whether, and what form of, legalization even makes it to the ballot.

The Proposals' Salient Characteristics

The details of legalization proposals are important. Among the key distinctions to make with respect to the 2012 proposals is between the categories of: (1) *Repeal Only,* (2) *Repeal & Regulate,* or (3) *Repeal & Delegate.* Table I classifies the 17 proposals into these categories.

Table I: Categories of the 2012 Proposals

Repeal Only	*Repeal & Regulate*	*Repeal & Delegate*
• CA Cannabis Hemp and Health Initiative	• CA Regulate Marijuana Like Wine Act	• CA Repeal Cannabis Prohibition Act
• MI Constitutional Amendment To End Marijuana Prohibition	• CO Regulate Marijuana Like Alcohol Act	• MO Constitutional Amendment to Art. IV
• MT Proposal	• WA State Initiative 502	• OR Cannabis Tax Act
• OR Initiative Proposal 24	• MA Bill H-1371	• NE Initiative, Prop XIX
	• WA HB 1550	• NH HB 1705

Repeal Only proposals simply repeal the state's prohibition against marijuana—except perhaps for use by minors or while operating a vehicle. These proposals can be quite short; the proposed Constitutional Amendment to End Marijuana Prohibition in Michigan is only 88 words.[8]

Repeal & Regulate proposals not only repeal state prohibition, they also design a framework for the state to regulate the legal marijuana market. These proposals can be quite detailed. For example, WA I-502 runs into 62 pages (Holcomb 2012). Typical provisions include designating the market regulator, establishing taxation and fee structures, detailing the licensing process, and setting limits on personal possession amounts. Some declare a regulatory scheme modeled after alcohol or tobacco; some discuss workplace use rules, driving under the influence regulations, and/or specify penalties for violations of the regulatory framework. Most ban marijuana smoking in public areas. Many distinguish home cultivation from commercial production, allowing

---

[8] The text, in its entirety, reads: "For persons who are at least 21 years of age who are not incarcerated, marihuana acquisition, cultivation, manufacture, sale, delivery, transfer, transportation, possession, ingestion, presence in or on the body, religious, medical, industrial, agricultural, commercial or personal use, or possession or use of paraphernalia shall not be prohibited, abridged or penalized in any manner, nor subject to civil forfeiture; provided that no person shall be permitted to operate an aircraft, motor vehicle, motorboat, ORV, snowmobile, train, or other heavy or dangerous equipment or machinery while impaired by marihuana" (Committee for a Safer Michigan 2012).

users to grow a limited number of plants for personal consumption without being licensed, but prohibiting them from selling.

The proposals vary in terms of how carefully the details are thought through. For example, most state that driving under the influence of marijuana would remain illegal, but do not define "under the influence" nor specify the type of test to be administered. (Marijuana is different from alcohol; impairment—as opposed to past use—is difficult to measure accurately, which one referee notes is itself a concern with legalization). WA I-502 is unusually precise in this regard, stating that the THC level determined from a blood test must not exceed 5.0 nanograms per milliliter for those 21 or older, and that minors may not have any marijuana in their system whatsoever. Some who favor legalization generally nonetheless oppose WA I-502 because of the likelihood that medical marijuana users will routinely exceed that threshold.

Repeal & Delegate proposals are similar to *Repeal & Regulate* in that they also plan for a state regulatory structure, but they do not themselves specify the regulations. Rather, they delegate that responsibility to the state legislature (Nebraska Proposition XIX), an existing state agency (Department of Revenue for New Hampshire HB 1705; Health and Senior Services in Missouri), or a newly created "Cannabis Commission" (OCTA; CA Repeal Cannabis Prohibition Act). The proposals also vary widely in how well-written they are; some are carefully crafted, but others neglect important issues or are ambiguous in seemingly unintentional ways. For example, Oregon's IP-24 repeals criminal and civil sanctions for "private personal use, possession or production of marijuana." It is not immediately obvious whether "private personal" is meant to modify "use" or "use, possession, or production"—a distinction of considerable consequence.

Proposals vary in their response to the reality of continued federal and international prohibition. Massachusetts HB 1371 calls for creation of a Cannabis Control Authority only after *federal* marijuana prohibition is repealed. By contrast, the OCTA specifies that a state agency (the to-be-created Oregon Cannabis Commission) would sell cannabis through state stores. State employees operating these stores would be in direct violation of the federal Controlled Substances Act. The OCTA also defines itself as "a scientific experiment,"[9] perhaps as a nod to the international drug control conventions' allowing exceptions for experiments.

Some proposals are naïve about the potential power of the commercial interests that would be created.[10] The seven-person Oregon Cannabis Commission charged with regulating the cannabis industry would be comprised of five commissioners to be "elected at large by growers and processors" and just two appointed by the Governor. Building a super-majority of industry representatives into the regulatory body of that industry practically guarantees the sort of regulatory capture that has been problematic in diverse industries, dating from railroads under the old Interstate Commerce Commission and arguably including alcohol today.[11]

---

[9] In particular, "a scientific experiment" by the people of the state of Oregon to lower the misuse of, illicit traffic in, and harm associated with cannabis."

[10] This is a particular concern of organizations such as But What About the Children.

[11] By way of contrast, Massachusetts SB 1371 would have the governor appoint three, and the president of the senate and speaker of the house each appoint two of its seven-member Cannabis Control Authority.

Table II[12] summarizes key provisions of CO-RLA, OCTA, and WA I-502, which are on the 2012 ballot, and also of CA-RMLW, the California proposal that garnered the most signatures.

Table II: Comparison of Three Initiatives[13]

Policy		CA Regulate MJ Like Wine	CO Regulate MJ Like Alcohol	WA I-502	OR Cannabis Tax Act
Personal Use	Personal possesion limit	No limit	1 oz.	1 oz.	Not specified
	Restrictions on personal cultivation (plants allowed)	24+ (mature plants)	6 (3 or fewer mature)	0 (though 15 for registered medical marijuana patients)	Not specified
Regulation	Regulatory body name	Alcohol Beverage Control (ABC)	Department of Revenue	State liquor control board	Oregon Cannabis Commission (OCC)
	Body responsible for quality control	Not specified	Third party with valid license	Independent third party	Independent third party
	Allows for state-run stores	No	No	No	Yes
	Explicitly forbids cooperation with federal law enforcement on marijuana related cases	State is "ordered to protect and defend all provisions of this Act from any and all challenges or litigation, whether by persons, officials, cities, counties, the state or federal governments."	No	No	Attorney General required to "vigorously defend" the act and propose and urge the removal of federal impediments to the act.
Protection of Minors	Penalty to providing marijuana to minors	Up to $2,500	For over 2 oz: Class 4 Felony, 2-6 years in prison and up to $2,000.	For 18-20: Class C Felony (Up to 5 years in prison and a $10,000 fine) For Under 18: Class B Felony (Up to 10 years in prison and a $10,000 fine)	Sale: Class B Felony (up to $250,000 fine and/or 10 years in jail) Gratuitous provision: Class A Misdemeanor (up to $6,250 fine and/or 1 year jail)
	Penalty for possessing marijuana as a minor	Up to $2,500	For over 2 oz.: Misdemeanor, 3-12 months in prison and $250-$1,000 fine.	For first offense, under 40g: Misdemeanor (Up to 90 days in jail and a $250 fine)	$250
Taxation	Taxation rate	Similar to wine	15% on retail sales	25% (at each level)	N/A. OCC would set state store prices.
	Revenue use	Not specified	$40 million to public Schools	Various state agencies	State general fund and various state agencies

CO-RLA and WA I-502 share features. Both limit (unlicensed) personal possession to one ounce and contain provisions concerning impaired driving and sale to minors. Both earmark tax revenues to popular causes. For example, CO-RLA directs that the first $40 million in revenue the excise tax captures would be directed to a public school

---

[12] We are indebted to Becca Gillespie for creating this table.

[13] CO-RLA and WA I-502 make no changes to current state penalties regarding minors. The descriptions of the penalties above highlight key points but should not be viewed as comprehensive; for a full understanding, direct consultation of the state laws is advised.

capital construction fund.[14] Yet, there are salient differences. WA I-502 assigns the State Liquor Control Board to regulate the industry while CO-RLA assigns that function to the Department of Revenue. They also differ with respect to specificity. WA I-502 includes protections such as limiting a licensee's operation to a single, fixed location and imposing a range of restrictions on the operation of retail stores. CO-RLA does not include such protections, but its supporters believe the Department of Revenue has been effective at regulating medical marijuana and that it is reasonable to believe it will be comparably effective in regulating the legal, non-medical industry.

As a *Repeal & Delegate* proposal, OCTA leaves several important provisions, including maximum amounts allowed for personal possession, undetermined. And while it specifies no tax rate, the state-stores would sell non-medical marijuana at a substantial markup over what they paid the licensees to produce it, which OCTA anticipates would produce net revenues for the state.

Federal Responses and Market Impacts

The following discussion considers ways in which the federal government may respond to state legalization, and how these varying responses may lead to different outcomes. Space and data limitations preclude a full benefit-cost analysis, but readers should keep in mind three distinct categories of costs: (1) Costs of regulation and enforcement. (2) Costs associated with marijuana use, including direct health effects and outcomes such as dependence and impaired driving. (3) Collateral consequences of black markets, which are determined in no small measure by who profits from production and sale—criminals, conventional businesses, or the state itself. A general theme is that the federal response will create tradeoffs among these categories of costs; no option minimizes all three simultaneously. The aim here is just to help readers understand the complexity of the choices, not to suggest what course of action is best.

Arrest Risk

A state may legalize marijuana for adults, perhaps as soon as November 2012, but marijuana would remain illegal at the federal level, and the federal government would probably not stand idly by. The response to medical marijuana is instructive. President Obama flatly rejected legalization at the recent Cartagena summit (Calmes 2012), and some media sources describe the Obama administration as even harsher than George W. Bush was in cracking down on large-scale medical marijuana dispensaries (Dickinson 2012). Nevertheless, the federal government may be reluctant to run roughshod over programs directly endorsed by the voters at the ballot box, and the federal government continues *not* to intervene in state-sanctioned medical marijuana distribution except for large-scale operations and/or those that violate (its reading of) state law.

---

[14] WA I-502 takes the strategy to heart, earmarking funds for the Department of Social and Health Services, the Department of Health, the University of Washington, Washington State University, the state basic health plan trust account, the Washington State Health Care Authority, and the Office of the Superintendent of Public Instruction.

Furthermore, while federal agents would clearly retain the power to arrest anyone anywhere in the United States for any marijuana violation—even possession by someone with a medical marijuana card—it is equally clear that federal agencies lack the resources to fill in for the removal of all state and local enforcement.

In 2010, state and local law enforcement made 97% of the more than 800,000 marijuana sales and possession arrests nationwide (FBI Uniform Crime Report 2012). The majority of those arrests were for possession, and it seems unlikely that the federal government could, or would want to, assume the burden of deterring individual marijuana users.

The situation for sellers is similar, albeit less extreme. State and local agencies account for roughly 90% of marijuana sales and distribution arrests away from the Southwest Border; federal prosecutors often only accept cases involving hundreds of pounds of marijuana, not just one or two pounds, let alone one or two ounces or joints. Figure I shows the total number of marijuana *sales* arrests per state for some states considering legalization, and the share of those arrests made by the Drug Enforcement Administration (DEA). The far-left column shows the total number of marijuana arrests the DEA made nationwide.

Figure I: Marijuana Sales Arrests by State

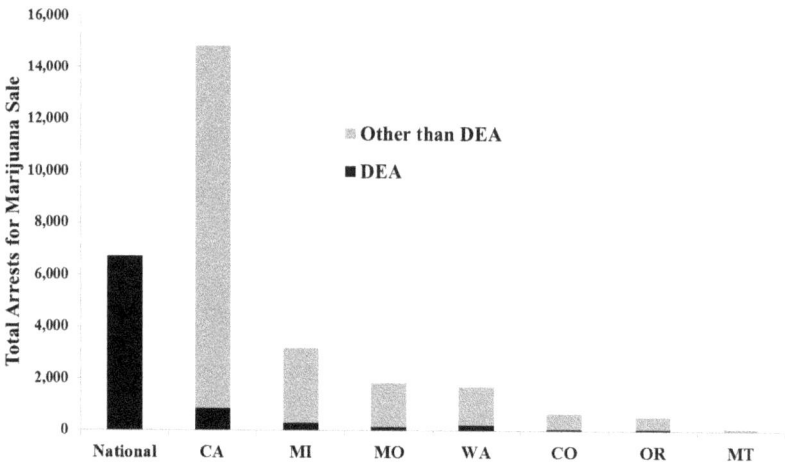

Sources: State totals from drugscience.org; DEA figures from DEA (personal communication).

The figure suggests that if the DEA or other federal enforcement agencies do not reallocate resources, legalization in any given state will lead to a roughly 90% drop in arrests of marijuana sellers in that state, presumably with a greater than 90% drop for lower-level sellers and a less than 90% drop for higher-level distributors.

Second, the DEA's ability to fill in for "missing" sales arrests varies with the size of the state. State and local enforcement agencies in California make more sales arrests than the DEA does *nationwide*, not just in California. For states like Washington the DEA could apparently make up for the missing marijuana sales arrests, but doing so with the existing resources would noticeably reduce enforcement intensity elsewhere. By contrast, Montana in a typical year has fewer than 100 marijuana sales arrests; if Montana were the only state to legalize, it would be entirely possible for the DEA to prevent any reduction in enforcement risk for sellers.

Additional Federal Strategies

Strategic options for the federal response to *Repeal Only* legalization are limited. The main question is how much additional enforcement to allocate to the state. There are many particulars. What kind of enforcement? Should redirected enforcement be solo or cooperate with police in surrounding states? What are the targets? Should it be across the board or with particular intensity at those who advertise or fail to label accurately? But, the question boils down to: How much enforcement?[15]

However, if a state passes a *Repeal & Regulate* form of legalization, the federal government can choose among a complicated set of responses, each carrying its own drawbacks and benefits. Potential options include: sending letters to landlords, banks, and other business owners threatening them with asset seizure for cooperating with illegal activities, preempting parts or all of state laws, and/or seizing tax revenues collected from marijuana commerce. The same general strategies are also relevant to *Repeal & Regulate* proposals, although how the particulars work out depend on future choices of the regulatory body to which authority is delegated.

Letters

U.S. Attorneys have sent letters informing landlords who rent to medical marijuana dispensaries that their tenants are violating federal law, and threatening to confiscate their property unless they evict their tenants. Landlords typically comply. The cost to the government of inducing such "third party policing" is minimal (Mazerolle and Ransley 2006), so these interventions can be highly cost-effective for the government, albeit limited to instances in which the marijuana dispensary is operating from a fixed storefront.

There are reports of similar letters being sent to banks, warning them to cease doing business with marijuana dispensaries or risk losing their charters, access to FDIC insurance, etc., on the grounds that they are violating federal money-laundering laws (Frichtel 2012).

Of course U.S. Attorneys could also send letters to landlords renting to marijuana sellers in a *Repeal Only* state if those sellers tried to operate flagrantly from a storefront. However, while *Repeal Only* proposals remove all penalties for production, sale, and possession, they impose no positive obligations, such as obtaining a license or operating out of a fixed location. Legal operations under *Repeal Only* proposals could remain covert then, making it hard for attorneys to figure out where to send the letters.

---

[15] We simplify. Nothing limits the options for the federal response to marijuana-specific policies. Under the Reagan Administration, states raised their minimum alcohol purchase ages in part in response to the Administration's threats to withhold a portion of their federal highway dollars. The federal government might similarly withhold highway dollars, or some other funding stream, from states that legalize. Retroactive punishment may or may not be useful; voter propositions can be notoriously hard to repeal. Pre-emptive creation of a "poison pill" before legalization passes might be more effective, but that would require strategic thinking about a possible future "threat", not just reacting to front-burner issues.

Preemption
The Preemption Doctrine stems from the supremacy clause of the Constitution (Article VI, clause 2). It holds that federal law trumps state law when there is conflict between the two. The Controlled Substances Act (CSA) is federal law and contains an explicit provision on preemption of state and local laws. Preemption occurs when "there is positive conflict between [the CSA and] state [or local] law so that the two cannot consistently stand together" (21 U.S.C. Section 903).

State and federal laws can be incongruous without meeting the positive conflict test. Medical marijuana provides an instructive example. The U.S. Supreme Court clearly established that federal marijuana law trumps state or local law by upholding the federal government's right to enforce marijuana prohibition even in states that had legalized medical marijuana (*Gonzales v. Raich* 2005). Nonetheless, *Gonzales v. Raich* does not nullify state medical marijuana laws; those laws continue to function at the state level. Imagine state statutes or regulations require a marijuana dispensary to pay an annual licensing fee; the state can punish dispensaries that do not comply.

We shall not attempt to ascertain exactly how courts would apply preemption to state-level legalization proposals; that analysis is better left to legal scholars. However, a lay reading suggests that the proposals vary in their level of conflict with the CSA. Generally, *Repeal Only* proposals steer clear of conflict since they merely cancel the state's prohibition. Indeed, New York State repealed its prohibition of alcohol in 1923 despite continued federal prohibition, and other states subsequently followed suit (Caulkins et al. 2012).

At the other extreme, certain provisions in some *Repeal & Regulate* proposals conflict so directly that a federal challenge would seem almost certain to prevail. An example mentioned above is OCTA's mandate that state-run stores sell marijuana. Another is the California Cannabis Hemp & Health Initiative's stipulation that "Any person who threatens the enjoyment of these provisions is guilty of a misdemeanor." A provision that would make it illegal for DEA agents to enforce the CSA would presumably be preempted.

Many other provisions might occupy some intermediate ground. For example, some proposals have state agencies setting quality standards; others would have state employees actively engaged in the process of testing quality. The latter requires physically possessing the marijuana. Possession is generally illegal under the CSA, but there is an exception for government employees acting in their official capacities (e.g., to protect local police when they seize illegal drugs). Our guess, and it is only a guess, is that licensing would not be preempted. Licensing is a traditional state function, and licensing market participants might be seen as comparable to issuing medical marijuana cards. Thus far, state courts have held that medical marijuana laws do not frustrate the purposes of the CSA because there is no "positive conflict." As Oregon's Supreme Court ruled:

> It is not physically impossible to comply with both the [state medical marijuana law] and the federal Controlled Substances Act. To be sure, the two laws are logically inconsistent; state law authorizes what federal law prohibits. However, a person can comply with both laws by refraining from any use of marijuana (*Emerald Steel Fabricators, Inc. v. Bureau of Labor and Industries* 2010).

Other state courts have ruled against the application of preemption to medical marijuana because regulation of medical practices is a common state function (*County of San Diego v. San Diego NORML* 2008). Federal courts have not yet ruled on the preemption question regarding medical marijuana laws (The court has made clear, e.g., in *Gonzales v. Raich,* that the federal government can enforce federal marijuana laws in states with medical marijuana laws; that is a different question than whether federal law preempts the state's laws or regulations).

By extension, collecting fees from licensees might also survive; after all, some states already collect such fees from medical marijuana cardholders. It is unclear whether the federal government will preempt taxation. On the one hand, jurisdictions such as the City of Oakland have successfully assessed and collected marijuana-specific taxes on medical marijuana. On the other hand, even if general taxation does not provoke preemption, certain earmarks that further promulgate marijuana activity might. For example, the California Cannabis Hemp & Health Initiative's earmark that 50% of tax revenues be dedicated to "research, development, and promotion of industrial and medical hemp industries" may be considered to positively conflict with the CSA.

Seizure of Tax Revenues

The claim that legalization can ease state fiscal woes has been an important attraction, perhaps particularly for median or swing voters (cf., Kilmer et al. 2010a). Many proposals include tax provisions of diverse levels and forms. New Hampshire SB 1775 would set the tax at $45 per ounce, while Missouri would place an upper limit on taxes of no more than $100 per pound (about $6 per ounce). Those two taxes differ in amount but both would be assessed per unit weight. Others, including CO-RLA and WA I-502, are expressed as a percent of value (ad valorem). Massachusetts HB 1371 taxes THC rather than marijuana by assessing a tax of $10 per percentage point of THC per ounce. (For example, marijuana that was 5% THC by dry weight would be taxed at $50 per ounce.)

The tax component of legalization proposals could be fragile. Even if tax clauses are not preempted, the federal government could still seize tax revenue under federal money laundering statutes. The federal government has not done this with respect to medical marijuana taxes yet. The City of Oakland collected $1.4 million in taxes from marijuana dispensaries in 2011 and the State of Colorado $5 million (Cooper 2012). But that it has not seized these revenues in the past does not mean it could not in the future.

Double-Edged Swords

The aggressiveness with which the federal government responds to a *Repeal & Regulate* legalization scheme would influence many facets of the legal market including changes in price and use, who the suppliers are, the effectiveness of state regulation, and tax revenue collection.

Several variables factor into the prevalence and intensity of marijuana use. For example, users can be deterred by social stigma or fear of future negative effects whether health-related or not. But the government exerts two additional restraints on use: enforcement pressure and regulatory structures.

Enforcement pressure increases the cost of illegal marijuana through "structural consequences of product illegality" (Reuter 1983) and the "risks and prices" mechanism (Reuter and Kleiman 1986). "Structural consequences of illegality" are impediments to efficient business operations that the requirement to produce and move products underground imposes on suppliers. The "risks and prices" mechanism refers to the fact that suppliers take risks by providing illegal goods, and expect compensation for taking those risks. Higher prices tend to suppress marijuana consumption (Grossman 2005; Pacula 2010), just as they do for consumption of many other goods (for a thorough explanation, see Caulkins and Reuter 2010).

Regulatory structures can also partially restrain use. This is clearest with respect to taxes, which—if they are successfully collected[16]—drive up retail price and so, push down consumption; that is why the public health community tends to support raising tobacco and alcohol taxes. Some proposals include additional restraints. Massachusetts SB 1371 includes language limiting sales to licensed, enclosed premises, with customers restricted to adults who are not visibly intoxicated. Retailers would be required to post prominent warnings that cannabis consumption may impair driving and cause health problems; vending machine sales would be prohibited; licensees would not be allowed to advertise; and the Commission would have ongoing responsibility for adjusting the laws to prevent abuse and evasion. Furthermore, regulatory structures can also mitigate harm for specific groups, such as protecting minors from the effects of advertising.

At least in theory both federal enforcement and state regulatory structures could help mitigate the legalization-induced increase in use. However, resource-constrained federal enforcement agencies seeking to dismantle a state's legal market may find these regulatory structures and/or regulated suppliers to be among their easiest targets.

Therefore, federal enforcement can be a double-edged sword. Officials would have to decide between intensifying enforcement pressure to soften the price decline and thereby limit the increase in use, or tolerating the legal market so that state regulatory structures can curb abuse and misuse.

To be more specific, it would be relatively easy—not easy, but relatively easy—to shut down licensed bricks-and-mortar marijuana stores by sending threatening letters from U.S. Attorneys to landlords, banks, insurers, and other companies that a legitimate retail establishment depends on to operate. But that would push the trade back to unregulated suppliers who—after state and local police have ceased enforcement—could operate with relative impunity for a while, unless the federal government mustered the resources to substitute for state and local enforcement.

Likewise, if state taxation and/or regulations were preempted, but the federal government did not otherwise increase its enforcement efforts, then we might expect a larger price decline than if the federal government did not interfere at all, but a smaller one than if it had interfered more heavily and directly.

Realistically, the regulatory structures contemplated by the 2012 proposals—even by Massachusetts SB 1317— are not very potent when it comes to restraining use. Likewise, there are limits on the extent to which enforcement can drive up prices (Caulkins and Reuter 2010). A scenario in which federal enforcement is lighter than current enforcement, and another in which the federal government significantly increases its level of enforcement, might involve noticeable but not overwhelming differences in levels of

---

[16] This is a legitimate concern in itself. See "Tax Collection and Evasion" section of this paper.

use. That is, either scenario might involve roughly comparable increases in consumption compared to the status quo.

However, the federal response could substantially affect who receives the dollars consumers spend on marijuana. If the federal government takes a hands-off approach, in effect respecting the will of the voters in the state that legalizes, then marijuana might—under at least some proposals—be just another product sold from the shelves of convenience stores. Or, marijuana might be sold in dedicated marijuana-only stores, akin to state liquor stores. Either way, the marijuana industry would be legitimate, with profits going to businesspeople similar to those who profit from the sale of other goods, including alcohol or cigarettes.

The federal government could also respond with a slight increase in enforcement, possibly by preventing marijuana businesses from obtaining loans or leasing fixed storefronts. In this scenario, retail might be dominated by smaller-scale entrepreneurs operating with modest capital investment, as do mobile food vendors ("food trucks"), farmers' market booths, or home delivery services like some dispensaries offer.

With still greater pressure, these smaller-scale licensed vendors might be replaced by unlicensed distributors who are not otherwise criminally involved, perhaps akin to the "$5 men" who hawk untaxed cigarettes in New York City's gray market (Shelley et al. 2007).

And, with a concerted effort, the federal government could make the structure of the marijuana industry look like marijuana in states without liberal medical marijuana laws, which is to say, it would be an underground activity whose revenues went primarily to professional criminals.

So the federal government's actions might have a real but modest effect on marijuana use and use-related harms, but a large effect on who receives the profits from selling marijuana and, hence, on the amount of collateral damage the selling creates.

Having touched on the topics of a price decline and consumption increase, the next section discusses these topics more thoroughly.

Characteristics of a Legal Marijuana Market

Prices in States that Legalize

It is generally recognized that marijuana prices will fall after legalization because the prices users currently pay are extremely high relative to what it would cost to produce, process, and transport marijuana if these activities were legal. Any resulting price decline would tend to increase both the number of users and the amount users consume (Grossman 2005; Pacula 2010; Kilmer et al. 2010a).

Production costs would be almost negligible with national legalization that allowed true farming of marijuana. Outdoor cultivation can annually yield on the order of 2,000 pounds of dry, high-grade marijuana per acre at a growing cost likely to be on the order of $2,000 to $20,000 per year. Thus, even after factoring processing and distribution costs, nationwide legalization could cut retail price to a few dollars or a few tens of dollars per pound, as opposed to wholesale sinsemilla prices of several thousand dollars per pound today (Geiringer 2009b; Caulkins et al. 2012).[17]

---

[17] Though we note that farmgate prices for marijuana have been dropping in the emerald triangle (Brand 2012).

State-level legalization is more complicated because of uncertainty about the federal response and its effect on the dominant production modality. Kilmer et al. (2010a) developed quantitative business models to project the per-pound cost for growing high-grade marijuana and estimated it to be $30 for a farm, $70–$215 for a greenhouse, and $200–$400 for a dedicated 1,500 square foot "grow house."[18]

Even though production costs are lower for farms and greenhouses, Kilmer et al. guessed that grow houses would dominate because production would still be illegal under federal law. Farms and greenhouses would be too easy for federal enforcement to detect and seize.

We adapted Kilmer et al.'s model to estimate production costs and resulting legal prices in California under CA-RMLW, in Colorado under CO-RLA, and in Washington under WA I-502 (OCTA is excluded from this analysis because it does not specify a tax rate). Our estimates are broadly consistent with those of Kilmer et al. (2010a), but are a little lower for grow houses in Colorado ($175–$340 per pound) and Washington ($160–$330 per pound) than for California because of lower costs of rent and electricity.[19]

The wholesale and retail prices are inflated above these production cost estimates by: (1) the wholesale price markup, (2) the retail price markup, (3) the usual state and local sales tax, and (4) the proposal's excise tax. For California and Colorado we use Kilmer et al.'s (2010a) 25% wholesale and 33% retail markups, Drenkard's (2012) average combined state and local sales tax of 8.11% for California and 7.44% for Colorado, and the excise taxes proposed in California and Colorado.[20]

The corresponding estimate for WA I-502 is complicated by its unusual tax structure. WA I-502 imposes a 25% excise tax at each of three points along the supply-chain: first, when the producer sells to the processor; second, when the processor sells to the retailer; and third, when the retailer sells to the consumer. Given this legally required supply-chain and tax structure, we include also a 15% distributor markup as a proxy for the processor markup (Beaman and Johnson 2006), and use Drenkard's average combined state and local sales tax in Washington of 8.8%.

Table 3 shows the resulting estimates for prices in each state, using the midpoints of the grow house production cost estimates. It is important to note that these price estimates would pertain to the new steady-state market conditions. It is not clear how long it would take the industry to expand enough to push prices down to these levels. Prices would not fall overnight; the full decline might well take five or more years.

---

[18] A "grow house" in this context is a residence used strictly for marijuana cultivation. The producers install growing equipment including lights, a watering system, and other components depending on the complexity of the operation.
[19] Kilmer et al. estimated rent in California would cost around $35,000 per year versus only $24,000 per year in Colorado and $26,000 per year in Washington (Zillow Real Estate Market Reports 2012). Likewise, according to the Energy Information Administration, residential electricity costs 14.75 cents per kilowatt-hour in California, but only 11.04 cents in Colorado and 8.04 cents in Washington.
[20] CO-RLA specifies a retail excise tax of up to 15% on non-medical marijuana. CA-RMLW merely says that taxes and regulations similar "to the grape farming and wine industries... shall apply to marijuana" without explaining what marijuana tax would be similar to California's tax of 20 cents per gallon of wine. For this exercise, we consider an excise tax of 20 cents per one-eighth ounce of marijuana, a typical purchase weight, which would tax hours of intoxication at roughly similar rates.

Table 3: Long-Run Legal Price Estimates by State

	California	Colorado	Washington
Wholesale Price	$375 per pound	$320 per pound	$380 per pound
Retail Price	$560 per pound $35 per ounce	$520 per pound $33 per ounce	$980 per pound $60 per ounce

Wholesale prices per pound for (illegal) high-grade forms currently range from $3,000 to $4,500 in California, $2,500 to $4,500 in Colorado, and $2,000 to $5,000 in Washington (Narcotic News 2012). Corresponding retail prices per ounce are typically between $250 and $375. Even in Washington, with its price inflated by the compounding tax structure, the "best guesses" of legal prices are much lower than current prices.

Kilmer et al. (2010a) note that it is very hard to bound the magnitude of the resulting price-induced consumption increase because the anticipated price declines go beyond the support of the historical data. Further complicating matters is the fact that consumption also reacts to non-price factors, such as reduced social approbation, more consistent quality, and more convenient access. MacCoun (2010) estimates that non-price factors associated with California's Proposition 19 might have increased consumption by 5–50% above and beyond that which would stem from price effects alone.

Effects on Prices in Other States

The price declines and associated effects on consumption would not be limited to the state or states that legalized for two reasons: drug tourism and interstate smuggling.

As the Dutch experience suggests, if a state legalizes, it could receive an influx of drug tourists hoping to take advantage of the opportunity to legally purchase and openly use marijuana. There is no obvious way to project how common this would be, but to give some sense of the potential magnitude, Figure II shows the number of past-month marijuana users that live within a certain distance of the borders of Missouri or Colorado, two states that entertained legalization proposals in 2012 (although only Colorado's proposition made it on the ballot). As an aside, conventional sales taxes on gasoline, hotel rooms, and restaurant meals purchased by drug tourists in the state that legalized could be non-negligible compared with revenues the marijuana sales taxes generate themselves, particularly for CO-RLA which initially caps excise taxes at 15% and exempts medical sales. (One-quarter of Colorado's past-month users possess medical recommendations).

Figure II: Past-Month Users within 500 Miles of Missouri and Colorado

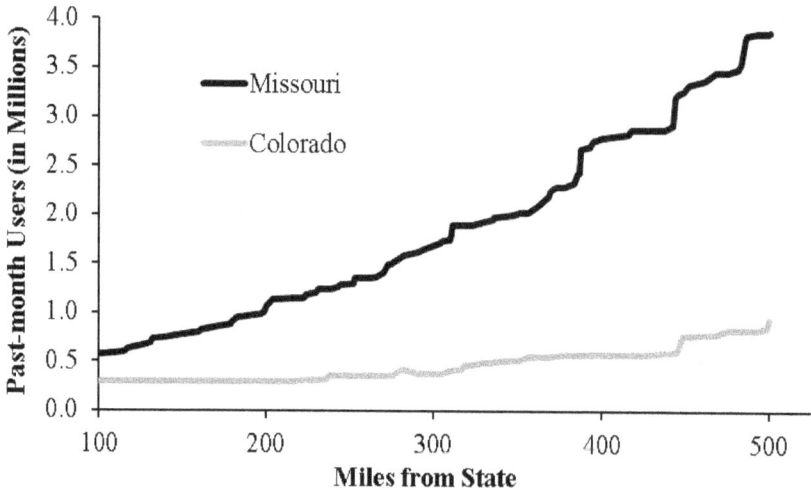

Legalization could also affect prices if marijuana traffickers choose to source marijuana from the state that legalizes, instead of from their current sources in Mexico or elsewhere. Inasmuch as marijuana traffickers are in the business for profit, one might expect them to gravitate to whatever "source zone" offered the product on the most favorable terms. As the previous section suggested, prices in a state that legalized could be quite low. Furthermore, there are obviously no international borders that must be crossed when smuggling marijuana from Colorado or Missouri to any other of the lower 48 states.

Based on seven different datasets, Caulkins and Bond (2012) estimated the wholesale price gradient when trafficking illegal marijuana within the United States to be about $400 per pound per one thousand miles. By adding this cost of illegal transport to the legal price that Kilmer et al. estimated, they found that marijuana produced legally in California and trafficked illegally across state lines could undercut current (quality-adjusted) prices in most other states.

We considered a similar scenario in which Colorado legalizes, using the cost estimates above, and confirmed this basic conclusion. Figure III illustrates the associated wholesale price decline estimated in each state, which could be substantial across the entire continental United States.

Figure III: Percent Price Decline by State Due to Spillover

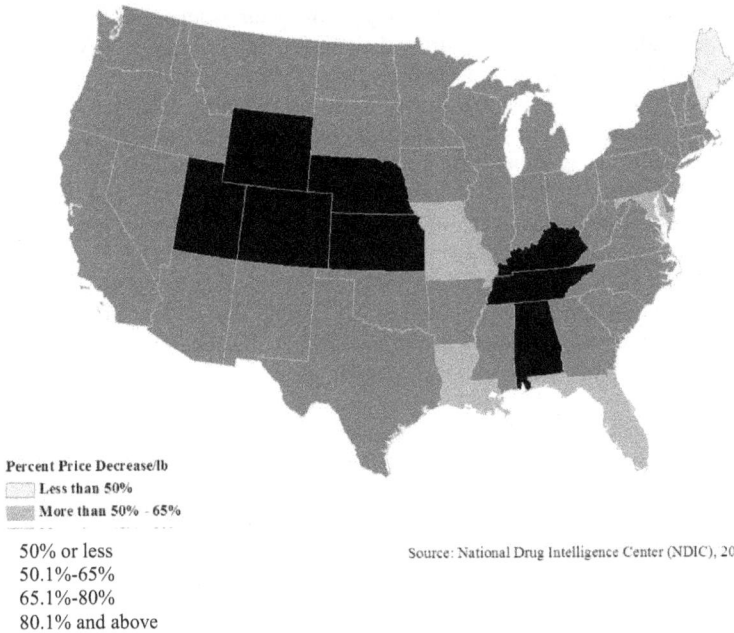

Percent Price Decrease/lb
  Less than 50%
  More than 50% - 65%

50% or less
50.1%-65%
65.1%-80%
80.1% and above

Source: National Drug Intelligence Center (NDIC), 2008.

Tax Collection and Evasion

Various groups have projected the potential tax revenues flowing from marijuana legalization. A typical, naïve approach multiplies the total value of the current market by the sales and/or excise tax rate. It is important to take such projections with a very large grain of salt, as we illustrate momentarily. Many proposals allocate tax revenues to various agencies, including those managing treatment services, public health and prevention efforts, and medical research. While such stipulations could theoretically offset some of the damages caused by increased drug use, it may be that in actuality, these agencies receive less funding than would be suggested by these naïve estimates.

Washington State's Office of Financial Management estimated that revenue derived from WA I-502 excise taxes would be about $450 million over its first full fiscal year (OFM 2012b). Underpinning this estimate is a before-tax retail price of $12 per gram, equivalent to $340 per ounce before tax, or $425 with the 25% excise tax. Even excluding sales taxes, this would be more than $150 higher than the current price per ounce of high-grade marijuana that users in Washington now report (Price of Weed 2012).

Taxes that raise prices above where the illegal market takes them should lead to concern about the possibility of tax evasion. Since marijuana already has a well-established underground market, evasion could take the form of simply continuing to buy from current sources. Alternately, licensed producers might produce additional quantities at the very low legal cost-of-production, but divert that excess to the tax-evading gray

85

market. This happens today in India, where poppy farmers licensed to produce for the pharmaceutical market sell excess production to the illegal market (Paoli et al. 2009).

A large enough tax might even negate the convenience of purchasing legal marijuana, and induce some users to grow their own at home legally. WA I-502 does not explicitly permit homegrown nonmedical cannabis though, so opting to grow one's own marijuana there instead of paying for it in stores would constitute illegal activity. However, medical marijuana patients and caregivers can grow up to 15 plants, and 15 plants can produce much more than one person's average annual consumption, even without considering the possibility of multiple plantings per year. Some proposals, like CO-RLA, do permit home growing, so choosing to grow at home in lieu of buying in a store amounts to legal tax avoidance.

CO-RLA provides users with another legal way to avoid paying taxes by exempting medical marijuana purchases from its excise tax. About one-quarter of Colorado's past-month users now have a medical recommendation. If obtaining medical marijuana approval is not difficult, then some additional users may register to obtain medical marijuana rather than purchase taxed non-medical marijuana.

Effective January 1, 2012 Colorado reduced the application fee for registry cards to \$35.[21] So someone who anticipated buying more than $35 \div 15\% = \$233$ worth of marijuana a year might find it more economical to obtain a medical marijuana card. Furthermore, inasmuch as it would not be difficult for one person with a card to buy on behalf of others, the breakeven consumption rate is probably better thought of as \$233 worth of marijuana consumed over the year by the individual and/or his or her close friends.

Taxing "Exports"

The previous section stressed threats to potential tax revenues, but the overall message is not pure pessimism so much as caution, bordering on agnosticism. From a budgetary perspective, there are upside scenarios, including collecting income taxes from previously illegal employment.

One upside scenario (from the legalizing state's budgetary perspective) is worth elaborating because of potential effects on incentives for other states to legalize, namely the possibility of taxing sales to residents of *other* states. This is easiest to imagine with drug tourism, as discussed above. However, it may even be possible with respect to marijuana dealers from other states who source their marijuana from the state that legalized. If there were no quantity limits on legal sales, then a marijuana dealer from another state might prefer to purchase legally—even if that meant paying a modest tax— in order to avoid the risk associated with making an illegal purchase.

This scenario—should it come to pass—might be particularly galling to the neighboring states. While the state that legalized would be collecting taxes that could offset any additional health costs associated with greater marijuana use, the surrounding states might face greater consumption (because marijuana will be cheaper) without any compensating tax revenues.

The neighboring states might become more inclined to consider legalization themselves, both to capture the "lost" tax revenues from their own citizens' consumption and also to "compete" for tax revenues from still other states. Figure IV illustrates a

---

[21] Patients with a household income that is 185% of the Federal Poverty Level or less qualify for a fee waiver.

scenario where Colorado legalizes first, but Michigan later follows, thereby competing with Colorado for any benefits of "serving" most of the market east of the Mississippi.

The desire to tax "exports" could initiate a "domino effect." The same can be said for other nontax benefits including job creation, a reduction in criminal justice expenditures, and simply demonstrating that what had previously seemed "unthinkable" might actually be feasible.

Figure IV: Hypothetical Implications of Michigan Responding to Colorado's Initial Legalization in Order to Compete for Exports to the Eastern United States

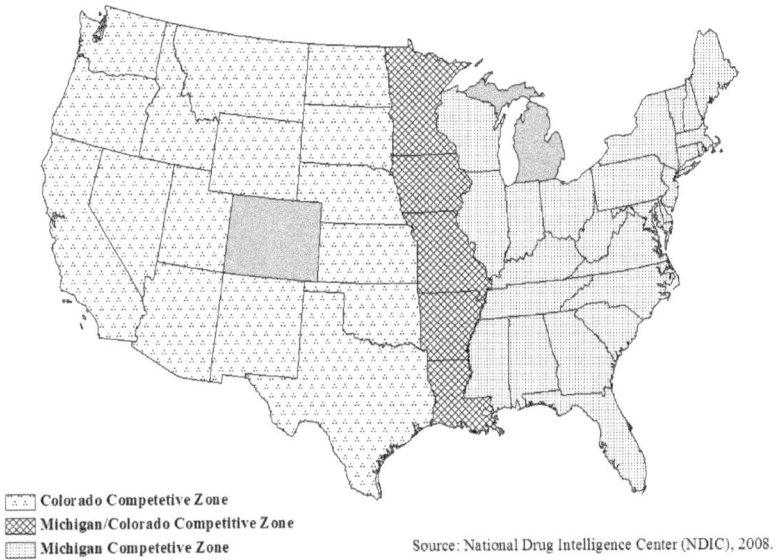

Colorado Competetive Zone
Michigan/Colorado Competitive Zone
Michigan Competetive Zone

Source: National Drug Intelligence Center (NDIC), 2008.

Hence, a single state legalizing may not be a stable equilibrium, of the sort that Nevada enjoyed with respect to casino gambling for over 40 years. If the pioneering state discovers that things go rather badly, whether because of higher than expected increases in abuse or because of punitive retaliation by the federal government, that state might reverse its legalization, restoring the status quo. On the other hand, if legalization runs more or less smoothly for the first state, perhaps particularly if it is able to tax exports, then other states might follow suit.

Conclusion: Lessons Learned

Perhaps the only safe conclusions with respect to marijuana legalization are that we live in interesting times, and that the future will make today's projections appear foolish in retrospect. However, a hedging strategy produces more interesting stock portfolios than discussion sections, so we tentatively offer the following "conclusions"; the quotations around the word "conclusions" are meant to convey that these statements are plausible and are supported by the analysis above, but they are by no means certainties.

State-Level Marijuana Legalization is a Real Possibility
Ten states considered 17 legalization proposals in 2012 with three voter propositions making it onto the ballot in states where polls suggest there is support from about half the population. It is important to stress that these proposals would not merely decriminalize or allow medical use. They would legalize (with respect to state law) commercial production without quantity limits. This would be unprecedented in a modern industrialized polity.

Even if legalization does not pass this year, the issue will likely return. New proposals will be revised in the light of lessons learned from 2012, in the same way that none of this year's proposals devolved regulatory authority to municipalities, one of the criticisms levied against Proposition 19 in 2010.

State-Level Legalization Is Not the Same as National Legalization
If a state legalized, federal prohibition would remain. State legalization of marijuana would produce very different outcomes from full national legalization.

State-Level Legalization Could Lead to Sharp Price Declines Nationwide
Kilmer et al. (2010a) established this finding with respect to California's Proposition 19 in 2010; parallel analysis of the prominent proposals in 2012 reaches similar conclusions. Production and distribution costs would fall sharply in the state that legalized. Over time, as the industry relocated and expanded, this would push down wholesale and retail prices in the state that legalized. Since smuggling within U.S. borders is not particularly expensive, the price decline would eventually be transmitted throughout the lower 48 states, leading to increases in use in each state.

Not All Legalization Proposals are Alike
Other than the basic reality of eliminating state and local enforcement (beyond regulatory compliance) the 17 proposals considered in 2012 were a heterogeneous lot. Commentators and voters might want to read the actual text of a legalization proposal before jumping to conclusions about effects or desirability.

The most salient distinction pertained to whether the proposal would merely end state and local enforcement (*Repeal Only*) or whether it would seek to substitute a regulatory structure, either directly (*Repeal & Regulate*) or by assigning that task to some agency (*Repeal & Delegate*).

"Repeal Only" Legalization Would Leave the Federal Government with Few Options
State and local agencies account for most marijuana enforcement. Except in small states, the federal government could not fill in for lost state and local efforts without greatly expanding the size and scope of federal enforcement. And *Repeal Only* proposals would not create a regulatory structure that the federal government could work with, attack, or sway.

"Repeal & Regulate/Delegate" Schemes Would Put the Federal Government in a Pickle

If the legalizing state tried to tax and tightly regulate the marijuana industry, the federal government could employ a variety of tools to disrupt or dismantle important parts of that regulatory structure.

However, while this might satisfy political demands to take action, it could exacerbate the increase in use by removing regulatory controls and preventing taxes from taking the edge off of the anticipated price decline. Furthermore, the federal response might have more effect on who receives the profits from the marijuana trade—whether they are conventional businesses or professional criminals—than it would on the size of the market or profits.

Legalization in Just One State May not be Stable

There is great uncertainty about how state-level legalization would turn out. If it turned out well—and perhaps particularly if the state could collect taxes on "exports" to other states—then other states might follow suit.

Concerns about Precedent Could Create Another Pickle

If legalization were not potentially "contagious," then a practical (practical in the literal, not political sense) federal response to one state implementing a reasonably designed *Repeal & Regulate* scheme might be to take a light-handed approach by only attempting to intercept smugglers carrying exports to other states.

However, such a lackadaisical response might encourage other states to also legalize, so some federal officials might be in the odd position of promoting actions that would make legalization worse in the first state, in order to "protect" other states from wanting to emulate it.

Implications for Public Health[22]

It is not possible to project with any precision the impact marijuana legalization will have on consumption (Kilmer et al. 2010a). However, it is a fact that that long-run prices will fall and that users—especially younger users—consume more when prices go down (Pacula 2010). Knowing this can motivate those interested or involved in developing programs and policies that seek to discourage drug abuse and misuse or to manage negative effects of marijuana use.

First, prevention curricula will need to be revised. It is generally accepted that prevention programs should be culturally congruent with the target population, and youth living in a state that has legalized will in a very literal sense be living in a different culture than that for which prevention programs were originally designed. Nevertheless, the increases in use are likely to be larger than what can be offset with prevention programs.

Second, there may be changes in demand for treatment. According to admissions data from the Treatment Episodes Data Set (TEDS), marijuana was the primary substance

---

[22] However tenuous are our conclusions about marijuana legalization, these implications for public health agencies should be taken with at least two more grains of salt. They are offered with the intent of provoking thought, not being anything like a final word on what is to be done.

of abuse for about one-third of instances in which the primary substance was not alcohol. Those 331,000 admissions were divided roughly equally between criminal justice referrals and other sources.[23] Perhaps adult criminal justice referrals (assuming juveniles are still referred) would shrink enough that treatment services would be able to handle an uptick in other referrals brought on by the increase in consumption. It would be Pollyanish or even wishful thinking not to anticipate *some* ramifications for treatment systems.

Third, it would become crucial to develop improved methods for roadside testing of marijuana-impaired driving.

Fourth, there may be both greater opportunity and greater need to investigate harm-reduction mechanisms of consumption. These mechanisms are analogous to broadly supported harm-reduction strategies for alcohol (such as designated driver programs) and HIV transmission for intravenously injected drugs (Babor et al. 2010), and their highly controversial counterparts for tobacco smoking (Stratton et al. 2001). For example, vaporizers do not combust marijuana, so users do not inhale combusted smoke, a potential risk factor for various lung diseases or other illnesses. Also, marijuana can be eaten, which is presumably the least harsh manner of consumption for a user's lungs, but its effects are much stronger when taken this way. When users accidentally ingest too much, they experience an overdose that may be benign on their physical body, but can be very distressing psychologically. Indeed, these negative experiences can last beyond the time the effects of the drug wear off and even uncover latent psychological problems. In this sense, harm reduction would entail instruction to users about drug administration and dosages.

Fifth, public health advocates may want to participate forcefully in fleshing out details concerning regulation. What matters is not just whether a state legalizes, but also *how* it legalizes. The devil, as they say, is in the details, and important choices concerning signage, public use, location of retail outlets, etc. will be in play as the regulatory regimes are sorted out.

Sixth, measures to help mitigate the increase in youth use may require a particularly forceful advocacy. Most proposals continue to ban use by those under the age of 21, but appear to imagine that a ban will itself take care of the issue. Some outside agencies, such as But What About the Children,[24] have begun to draw up criteria for "grading" various legalization proposals' performance at protecting youth from aggressive marketing by the newly legitimized marijuana industry.

Finally, any policy change of this importance should and will be evaluated. Indeed, WA I-502 earmarks funding for a cost-benefit evaluation by the Washington State Institute for Public Policy. Sketching the evaluation design is beyond the scope of this paper, but given the variation across states' proposals and the extent of anticipated spillovers across state borders, a panel data analysis that codes each state's legal status with simple binary variables would be inadequate, as has been the case of similar efforts to evaluate state decriminalization (Pacula et al. 2003).

---

[23] The state-specific proportions for Colorado, Oregon, and Washington are fairly similar to the proportions for the nation as a whole.

[24] http://www.butwhataboutthechildren.org/

References

Babor, Thomas, Jonathan Caulkins, Griffith Edwards, David Foxcroft, Keith Humphreys, Maria Medina Mora, Isidore Obot, Jurgen Rehm, Peter Reuter, Robin Room, Ingeborg Rossow, and John Strang. 2010. *Drug Policy and the Public Good*. New York: Oxford University Press.

Beaman, Jill A., and Aaron J. Johnson. 2006. *A Guide For New Manufacturers: Food Distribution Channel Overview*. Corvallis: Oregon State University. http://ir.library.oregonstate.edu/xmlui/bitstream/handle/1957/20443/em8921.pdf (accessed August 4, 2012).

Brand, Madeleine. 2012. "Has the bubble popped on California's Medical Marijana Market?" *The Madeleine Brand Show*, May 8. http://www.scpr.org/programs/madeleine-brand/2012/05/08/26386/has-the-bubble-popped-on-californias-medical-marij (accessed May 16, 2012).

The Bulletin of Cannabis Reform. 2009. "United States Marijuana Arrests (1982–2008)." http://www.drugscience.org/States/US/US_total.htm (accessed August 14, 2012).

Calmes, Jackie. 2012. "Obama Says Legalization Is Not the Answer on Drugs." *New York Times*, April 14. http://www.nytimes.com/2012/04/15/world/americas/obama-says-legalization-is-not-the-answer-on-drugs.html?_r=1 (accessed April 25, 2012).

Campaign to Regulate Marijuana Like Alcohol. 2012. "Amendment 54: The Regulate Marijuana Like Alcohol Act of 2012." http://www.regulatemarijuana.org/s/regulate-marijuana-alcohol-act-2012 (accessed August 15, 2012).

Cantu-Schomus, Andrea. 2012. "Secretary of State issues $65,000 penalty for pay per signature violation." April 23. http://www.oregonsosblog.us/tag/ballot-initiatives/ (accessed May 13, 2012).

Caputo, Michael R. and Brian J. Ostrum. 1994. "Potential Tax Revenue from a Regulated Marijuana Market: A Meaningful Revenue Source." *The American Journal of Economics and Sociology* 53 (4): 475-490.

Caulkins, Jonathan P., and Brittany M. Bond. 2012. "Marijuana Price Gradients: Implications for Exports and Export-Generated Tax Revenue for California After Legalization." *Journal of Drug Issues* 42 (1): 28-45.

Caulkins, Jonathan P., Angela Hawken, Beau Kilmer, and Mark A.R. Kleinman. 2012. *Marijuana Legalization: What Everyone Needs to Know*. New York: Oxford University Press.

Caulkins, Jonathan P. and Beau Kilmer. N.D. (forthcoming). "Criminal Justice Costs of Prohibiting Marijuana in California." In *Something's in the Air: Race and the Legalization of Marijuana,* eds. Katherine Tate, James Lance Taylor, and Mark Q. Sawyer. Routledge.

Caulkins, Jonathan P. and Peter Reuter. 2010. "How Drug Enforcement Affects Drug Prices". In *Crime and Justice – A Review of Research,* Vol. 39, ed. Michael Tonry. Chicago: University of Chicago Press, 213-272.

Clements, Tom. 2012. *"Strategic Plan Corrections Memo."* January 27. Colorado Springs: Colorado Department of Corrections. http://www.doc.state.co.us/sites/default/files/StrategicPlan%5B15%5D_Corrections%20 Memo%201-27-12.pdf (accessed August 4, 2012).

Colorado Department of Public Health and Environment. 2012. "Colorado Medical Marijuana Registry: Statistics." January 31. http://www.cdphe.state.co.us/hs/ medicalmarijuana/statistics.html (accessed April 2, 2012).

Committee for a Safer Michigan. 2012. "Constitutional Amendment to End Marihuana Prohibition in Michigan." The 2012 Michigan Ballot Initiative to End Marijuana Prohibition. https://help.repealtoday.org/ (accessed April 2, 2012).

Controlled Substances Act. 1970. 21 U.S.C. 13.

Cooper, Michael. 2012. "Cities Turn to a Crop for Cash." *New York Times*, February 11. http://www.nytimes.com/2012/02/12/us/cities-turn-to-a-crop-for-cash-medical-marijuana.html (accessed April 4, 2012).

County of San Diego v. San Diego NORML. 2008. 165 Cal.App.4th 798.

Dickinson, Tim. 2012. "Obama's War on Pot." *Rolling Stone,* February 16. http://www.rollingstone.com/politics/news/obamas-war-on-pot-20120216 (accessed July 23, 2012).

Drug Enforcement Administration (DEA). 2011. "DEA Staffing & Budget." United States Drug Enforcement Administration. http://www.justice.gov/dea/agency/staffing.htm (accessed May 16, 2012).

Drenkard, Scott. 2012. "State and Local Sales Taxes in 2012." Tax Foundation, April 14. http://taxfoundation.org/article/sales-tax-rates-major-us-cities (accessed August 4, 2012).

Emerald Steel Fabricators, Inc. v. Bureau of Labor and Industries. 2010. 348 Or. 159.

Frichtel, Robert. 2012. "Budding Pot Business Needs Legal Banking." *Bloomberg*, March 13. http://www.bloomberg.com/news/2012-03-13/budding-pot-business-needs-legal-banking-robert-frichtel.html (accessed April 4, 2012).

Gallup. 2012. "State of the States." July 23. http://www.gallup.com/poll/125066/ State-States.aspx (accessed July 23, 2012).

Gieringer, D. 2009a. "Benefits of marijuana legalization in California: California NORML Report". http://www.canorml.org/background/CA_legalization2.html (accessed August 4, 2012).

Geiringer, D. 2009b. "Testimony on the Legalization of Marijuana to the California Assembly Committee on Public Safety." October 28. http://norml.org/pdf_files/ AssPubSafety_Legalization.pdf (accessed August 4, 2012).

Gonzales v. Raich. 2005. U.S. 03-1454.http://www.law.cornell.edu/supct/html/03-1454.ZS.html/ (accessed July 23, 2012).

Grossman, Michael. 2005. "Individual Behaviours and Substance Use: The Role of Price." *Adv Health Econ Health Serv Re*s 16:15-39.

Hall, Wayne. 2001. *The Health and Psychological Effects of Cannabis Use.* Canberra, Australia: Commonwealth of Australia.

Harwood, H. 2000. *Updating Estimates of the Economic Costs of Alcohol Abuse in the United States: Estimates, Update Methods, and Data.* Rockville, MD: National Institutes of Health.

Herrnstein, R. J., George Lowenstein, Drazen Prelec and William Vaughan. 1993. "Utility maximization and melioration: Internalities in individual choice." *Journal of Behavioral Decision Making* 6: 149-185.

Holcomb, Allison. 2012. "Washington State Initiative Measure No. 502 (I-502)." Olympia, Washington: State of Washington Statute Law Committee. http://newapproachwa.org/content/initiative (August 4, 2012).

Johnson, Kirk. 2011. "Marijuana Push in Colorado Likens It to Alcohol." *New York Times*, January 26, 1.

Kilmer, B., J.P. Caulkins, R.L. Pacula, R.J. MacCoun, and P.H. Reuter. 2010a. *Altered State? Assessing How Marijuana Legalization in California Could Influence Marijuana Consumption and Public Budgets.* Santa Monica, CA: RAND Corporation.

Kilmer, Beau, Jonathan Caulkins, Brittany Bond, and Peter Reuter. 2010b. *Reducing Drug Trafficking Revenues and Violence in Mexico: Would Legalizing Marijuana in California Help?* Santa Monica, CA: RAND Corporation.

Kleiman, Mark. 1989. *Marijuana: Costs of Abuse, Costs of Control.* New York: Greenwood Press.

Kleiman, Mark. 1992. *Against Excess: Drug Policy For Results.* New York: BasicBooks.

MacCoun, Robert J. 2010. *Estimating the Non-price Effects of Legalization on Cannabis Consumption.* Santa Monica, CA: RAND Corporation.

MacCoun, Robert J. and Peter Reuter. 2001. *Drug War Heresies: Learning from Other Vices, Times, and Places.* Cambridge: Cambridge University Press.

Martin, Jonathan. 2012. "New Poll Shows Voters Split on Legalizing Marijunana." *The Seattle Times*, January 4, 1. http://seattletimes.nwsource.com/html/theblotter/2017157404_new_poll_shows_voters_split_on.html (accessed May 15, 2012).

Martin, Mickey. 2012. "CA Marijuana Initiatives: Statement of Unity– now show me the money." *The Puffington Host*, February 27, 1.

Mazerolle, Lorraine and Janet Ransley. 2006. "The Case for Third Party Policing." In *Police Innovation: Contrasting Perspectives*, eds. David Weisburd and Anthony Allan Braga. Cambridge UK: Cambridge University Press, 191-206.

Miron, J. A. 2010. *Budgetary Implications of Drug Prohibition.* Cambridge, MA: Harvard University.

Miron, Jeffrey A. 2012. "Making the Case for Legalization." *CNBC,* April 19: 1. http://www.cnbc.com/id/47071983 (accessed August 4, 2012).

Missouri Show-Me Cannabis Regulation. 2011. "The Initiative: Show-Me Cannabis Regulation." http://show-mecannabis.com/about/the-initiative/ (accessed August 15, 2012).

Montana Secretary of State. 2012. "Constitutional Initiative No. 110: A Constitutional Amendment Proposed by Initiative Petition." http://sos.mt.gov/Elections/2012/BallotIssues/CI-110.pdf (accessed April 2, 2012).

Morral, Andrew R., Daniel F. McCaffrey, and Susan M. Paddock. 2002. "Reassessing the Marijuana Gateway Effect." *Addiction* 97 (12):1493-1504.

Narcotics News. 2012. "Marijuana Prices in the USA. Narcotic News." http://www.narcoticnews.com/Marijuana-Prices-in-the-U.S.A.php (August 4, 2012).

Nebraska Secretary of State. 2011. "Legalization of Marihuana (Constitutional)." June 23. http://www.sos.ne.gov/elec/2012/pdf/Marijuana%20Initiative.pdf (accessed April 2, 2012).

National Drug Intelligence Center (NDIC). 2008. *National Illicit Drug Prices.* December. Washington, DC: U.S. Department of Justice. http://www.dare.com/home/DrugInformation/documents/32579p.pdf (accessed August 4, 2012).

Newport, Frank. 2012. "Record-High 50% of Americans Favor Legalizing Marijuana Use." *Gallup Politics*, October 17: 1. http://www.gallup.com/poll/150149/record-high-americans-favor-legalizing-marijuana.aspx (accessed April 2, 2012).

Office of National Drug Control Policy. 2004. *The Economic Costs of Drug Abuse in the United States, 1992-2002.* Washington, DC : Executive Office of the President.

Oregon Cannabis Tax Act 2012. 2012. "Oregon Cannabis Tax Act 2012." July 12. http://www.cannabistaxact.org/ (accessed August 4, 2012).

Pacula, R., MacCoun, R. Reuter et al. 2005. "What Does it Mean to Decriminalize Marijuana? A Cross-National Empirical Examination." *Advances in Health Economics and Health Services Research* 16:347-370.

Pacula, R.L. 2010. *Examining the Impact of Marijuana Legalization on Marijuana Consumption: Insights from the Economics Literature.* WR-770-RC. Santa Monica, CA: RAND Corporation.

Pacula, Rosalie L., Jamie F. Chriqui, and Joanna King. 2003. "Marijuana Decriminalization in the United States: What Does it Mean in the U.S.?" *National Bureau of Economic Research Working Paper Series* # 9690, May.

Paoli, Letizia, Victoria Greenfield, Molly Charles, and Peter Reuter. 2009. "The Global Diversion of Pharmaceutical Drugs. India: The Third Largest Illicit Opium Producer?" *Addiction*104:347-354.

Pratt, Calvin D., et al. 2012. "Bill Text: New Hampshire House Bill 1705." September 4. http://legiscan.com/gaits/view/349583 (accessed August 15, 2012).

Price of Weed. 2012. "Price of Weed: A Global Price Index for Marijuana." www.priceofweed.com (accessed April 2, 2012).

Public Policy Polling. 2012. "CO Voters Favor Assault Weapons Ban, Legal Pot, Civil Unions." August 8. http://www.publicpolicypolling.com/pdf/2011/PPP_Release_CO_080812.pdf (accessed August 13, 2012).

Reuter, Peter. 1983. Disorganized Crime: The Economics of the Visible Hand. Cambridge, MA: MIT Press.

Reuter, Peter and Mark Kleiman. 1986. "Risks and Prices: An Economic Analysis of Drug Enforcement." Crime and Justice: An Annual Review 9: 128-179.

Reuters. 2011. "Colorado: Legalization of Marijuana Makes the Ballot." New York Times, February 27, 1.

Robbe, Hindrick. 1998. "Marijuana's Impairing Effects on Driving are Moderate When Taken Alone but Severe when Combined with Alcohol." *Human Psychopharmacology: Clinical and Experimental* 13 (S2): S70-S78.

Roddy, Juliette, Caren L. Steinmiller, and Mark K. Greenwald. 2011. "Heroin Purchasing is Income and Price Sensitive." *Psychology of Addictive Behaviors* 25(2): 358–364.

Rolles, Stephen. 2010. "An Alternative to the War on Drugs. BMJ; 341. doi: 10.1136/bmj.c3360.

Room, Robin, Benedikt Fischer, Wayne Hall, Simon Lenton and Peter Reuter. 2010. *Cannabis: Moving Beyond the Stalemate*. Oxford: Oxford University Press.

Sensible California. 2012. "Repeal Cannabis Prohibition Act of 2012." http://repealcannabisprohibition.org/index.php?page=display&id=1 (accessed August 15, 2012).

Shelley, Donna, M. Jennifer Cantrell, et al. 2007. "The $5 Man: The Underground Economic Response to a Large Cigarette Tax Increase in New York City." *American Journal of Public Health* 97 (8): 1483.

State of California. 2012. "Governor's Budget Summary—2012-13." http://www.ebudget.ca.gov/pdf/BudgetSummary/SummaryCharts.pdf (accessed May 16, 2012).

Story, Ellen et al.; Common Wealth of Massachusetts. 2011. "House Bill 1371: An Act to regulate and tax the cannabis industry." Jan 19. http://www.malegislature.gov/Bills/187/House/H01371 (accessed August 15, 2012).

Stratton, Kathleen, Padma Shetty, Robert Wallace, and Stuart Bondurant, eds. 2001. *Clearing the Smoke: Assessing the Science Base for Tobacco Harm Reduction*. Washington, DC: National Academy Press.

Substance Abuse and Mental Health Services Administration. 2012. "Results from the 2010 National Survey on Drug Use and Health: Detailed Tables." http://www.samhsa.gov/data/NSDUH/2k10ResultsTables/NSDUHTables2010R/HTM/Sect5peTabs1to56.htm#Tab5.2A (accessed August 4, 2012).

Substance Abuse and Mental Health Services Administration (SAMHSA). 2012. *Treatment Episode Data Set—Admissions (TEDS-A)—Concatenated, 1992 to 2010)*. Ann Arbor, MI: Inter-university Consortium for Political and Social Research. http://www.icpsr.umich.edu/icpsrweb/SAMHDA/studies/25221 (accessed August 15, 2012).

Thompson, Ross A and Charles A. Nelson. 2001. "Developmental Science and the Media: Early Brain Development." *American Psychologist*. 56 (1): 5-15. *EBSCOHOST* (July 23, 2012).

United States Department of Justice Federal Bureau of Investigation. 2012. "Crime in the United States, by State, 2010." http://www.fbi.gov/about-us/cjis/ucr/crime-in-the-u.s/2010/crime-in-the-u.s.-2010/ (accessed August 4, 2012).

United States Energy Information Administration. 2011. "Average Retail Price for Bundled and Unbundled Consumers by Sector, Census Division, and State, 2010." November 14. http://205.254.135.7/electricity/sales_revenue_price/pdf/table4.pdf (accessed August 4, 2012).

Washington State Department of Revenue Office of Financial Management. 2012. "I-502 Worksheet." http://www.ofm.wa.gov/initiatives/2012/I-502_Worksheet.pdf (accessed August 14, 2012).

White, Helene Raskin; Hansell, Stephen. "Acute and Long-term Effects of Drug Use on Aggression from Adolescence into Adulthood." *Journal of Drug Issues* 28(4): 837-858.

"Zillow Real Estate Market Reports Local Information." 2012. http://www. zillow.com/local-info/ (accessed August 4, 2012).

Presidential Rhetoric and Policy Outcomes: The President and the American Struggle with Heroin Abuse

Philip Denis, MPA, *University of Georgia*
Andrew B. Whitford, PhD, *University of Georgia*

Introduction

For almost four decades, politicians and social commentators have claimed that the criminal justice system is overwhelmed by drug-related crimes (e.g., Parenti 2000; Wright 2003). Some argue that government intervention to control the trade in narcotics has not reduced the drug problem in the United States. This paper explains how the policy process has shaped the public provision of access to substance abuse treatment, specifically for heroin abuse, over the past four decades. Methadone maintenance is a way of reducing the harm heroin abuse causes to society (Massing 1998, 8). Potential benefits include removing addicts from the streets, decreasing the crime rate, and reducing the transmission of infectious diseases (e.g., HIV, hepatitis) (Holder 1998, 23).

Some of the major players in national policy for control of narcotics abuse have been the president, Congress, and an assortment of departments and agencies, along with issue networks created by concerned citizens (Whitford and Yates 2003, 995). The general approach to dealing with drug abuse is to imprison offenders (Austin and Irwin 2001, 5). There are few opportunities to receive treatment during incarceration, and even fewer after release, though this may change as more private organizations work with the federal government to increase access to treatment.

Using data drawn from the public statements of the president, we describe how presidents have addressed the role of treatment as a solution to the drug problem. Our data come from the *American Presidency Project* database.[1] Starting in the late 1960s and early 1970s, based on the number of mentions, presidents paid the most attention to this solution. During the mid-1970s, they paid little public attention to drug treatment as a social solution to the narcotics problem; this lack of attention persisted until the mid-1990s. Beginning in 2000, greater attention was once more given to the treatment solution (Massing 1998, 8).

The presidents led the process of selecting among legal mechanisms for dealing with the drug problem by shifting their attention. The president's emphasis on drug treatment in public policy, with a component of harm reduction, appears to surface during periods of high drug use and recede during years of declining use.

This essay describes how presidents have used their powers to shape a primary outcome in the American drug problem. We first describe the regulation of heroin and methadone maintenance as an approach to treatment. We follow this with a content analysis of how presidents have used the bully pulpit to shape the policy process.

The War on Drugs: Policy and Heroin Use

The American experience with opioid addiction dates to as early as the Civil War. Morphine, an opiate-based painkiller, was used on the battlefields in a war that saw the largest casualties in U.S. history (Kleber and Kellerman 1971, 379). It became the preferred painkiller before the Civil War with the development of the hypodermic syringe for injecting liquid solutions under the skin (Belenko 2001, 7). After the war, people could obtain opiates (and other pharmaceutical provisions

---

[1] Source: The American Presidency Project. n.d. http://www.presidency.uscb.

containing them) from physicians, over-the-counter at drugstores, grocery, and general stores, and by mail order (Brecher 1972, 3).

Federal laws restricting usage came in the early 1900s. President William Taft signed a federal law against importing or using opium for nonmedicinal purposes in 1909; President Woodrow Wilson signed the Harrison Act of 1914 (Belenko 2001, xxxii). Healthcare professionals were slow to recognize the problem of addiction. Only during World War I were laws passed to curtail the recreational use of morphine (Kleber and Kellerman 1971, 379).

In the early nineteenth century, heroin was acclaimed as the "most reliable drug at our command today to subdue cough" (Schleif 1901, 429). Many considered it harmless, with few side effects except for occasional "stupor, giddiness, and severe headache," clearly related to the "high" patients felt after consuming the medication (Schleif 1901). By the early 1900s, opium was known as "G.O.M.": God's own medicine (Brecher 1972, 8). But healthcare professionals also came to see heroin addiction as "a drug hunger or craving created by a metabolic deficiency as a result of opiate abuse" (Pearson 1970, 2571).

By the 1960s, Presidents John F. Kennedy and Lyndon Johnson focused on reducing the supply of drugs as the public demanded law enforcement and international efforts to curb illicit use. Law enforcement, which reduced the supply, often increased the market price per unit of opiates, and higher prices sometimes were a factor in the increase in property crime (Levine et al. 1976, 435). Addicts sought to finance their habits by selling stolen property, which often happened if substance abusers lived in deviant subcultures (Kleber and Kellerman 1971, 379).

The president often focused on increased crime rates. In the 1970s, President Richard Nixon increased federal funds for substance-abuse treatment as a harm-reduction approach to the problem. It was estimated that addicts needed to raise $45 per day to pay for their drugs and did so by committing an average of 1.5 crimes a week (Levine et al. 1976, 437). Analysts saw treatment as a solution to the crime problem. Over time, programs like needle exchange (in part to decrease AIDS/HIV infection rates) and opiate maintenance sought to minimize the harm of addiction and abuse by both individuals and communities. Substance abusers were offered opioid replacement therapy to reduce the crime associated with heroin use rather than to cure their addiction to opiates (Goode 1997, 81-83). Rather than punishment and law enforcement, the primary national drug control strategies were prevention, research, education, training, rehabilitation, and treatment (Musto 1987, 258).

In the late 1960s, scholars used data to compare increases in heroin use and increases in crime (DuPont and Greene 1973, 716). In 1969, Dr. Robert DuPont collected the urine samples of prisoners entering the Washington, D.C., jail system and discovered that 44 percent of the samples tested positive for opiates. This finding led Mayor Walter Washington to let DuPont treat prison-system addicts with methadone.[2] After Washington, D.C., and other major U.S. cities began reporting increasing heroin addiction, the media focused on the new class of heroin abusers: white, middle-class, suburban youths, and Vietnam vets (DuPont and Greene 1973, 716; Brecher 1972, 183-194); in Washington, D.C., alone, over 18,000 residents were reported affected by the use of heroin (DuPont and Greene 1973, 716). The federal Narcotics Treatment Administration (NTA) started testing inmates for drug abuse, with African Americans often over-represented in those inmate populations (DuPont and Greene 1973, 716).

Robert Dupont has said that this over-representation contributed to stigma associated with the government's use of methadone, to the point that communities often objected to the location of methadone treatment clinics and some users were unwilling to be treated.[3] One result was the introduction of "street methadone." This byproduct of an unregulated environment for methadone prescriptions led to the reselling of take-home prescriptions on the streets, which somewhat replaced the heroin supply in some cities. The response from treatment centers was to replace

---

[2] Frontline, "Frontline: Drug Wars: Interview with Dr. Robert DuPont," n.d., http://www.pbs.org/wgbh/pages/frontline/shows/drugs/interviews/dupont.html.
[3] Frontline, "Frontline: Drug Wars."

injection methadone with tablet or liquid forms, and to limit the use of methadone by clients outside of the prescribing clinics (DuPont and Greene 1973, 721).

In 1972, Nixon created the Special Action Office for Drug Abuse Prevention (SAODAP) and chose Dr. Jerome H. Jaffe to coordinate government programs and agencies for solving the drug problem. To implement Nixon's strategy to reduce the demand side of the drug problem, the federal budget for substance-abuse treatment increased from $59 million in the fiscal year 1970 to $462 million by the end of 1974 (Musto 1987, 258).

But the use of methadone maintenance in drug policy came to a halt with Nixon's resignation. The country turned again to law enforcement and punishment-based solutions. At the same time, there appears to have been a growing acceptance of the use of some drugs during the time periods of the Ford and Carter administrations (Musto 1987, 264). The Domestic Council Drug Abuse Task Force's 1977 *White Paper on Drug Abuse* discussed the possible legalization of less harmful drugs like marijuana (Musto 1987, 266). The House Select Committee on Narcotics Abuse and Control hearings in 1977 did not result in decriminalization, but they indicated a more tolerant attitude toward recreational use.

Drug policy received increased attention at the institutional level with the advent of President Ronald Reagan's "get tough" policies. The president's "War on Drugs" instituted longer jail sentences and stricter minimum sentence lengths for first-time offences (Austin and Irwin 2001, 7). A campaign of punishment and law enforcement followed, as some associated the heroin trade with violent crime and heroin use with the spread of disease, although studies documented no clear direct relationship between total property crime and addiction (Levine et al. 1976, 439). In retrospect, Reagan's policies increased the number of people in prison but had little impact on drug use (Conser et al. 2001, 121).

Federal spending on law enforcement increased after Reagan's two terms, as President George H.W. Bush used the new White House Office of National Drug Control Policy (ONDCP) to address drug-trade problems like those associated with cocaine and crack (Belenko 2001, 325). ONDCP centralized a number of important resources at the presidential level (Whitford and Yates 2009). We show below that the issue moved back off the presidency's agenda during Presidents Bill Clinton and George W. Bush's administrations. Federal spending remained relatively high during the early 1990s due to public perceptions about the importance of "diplomacy, coercion, money, and military force to stop the flow of drugs into the country" (Falco 1996, 121).

This describes the overall shape of presidential involvement in narcotics-use reduction policies. We next turn to a detailed description of harm reduction as a specific solution.

Harm Reduction: The Advent of Methadone Maintenance

German scientists created methadone during World War II (Methadone 1948, 90) as an alternative painkiller; Eli Lilly and Winthrop-Stearns developed it for use in the United States, partly through tests on federal prisoners at the Lexington, Kentucky, "Narcotics Farm" (Methadone 1948). The first experimental use of methadone maintenance treatment (MMT) was conducted in 1964 (Methadone Maintenance 1969, 1176). MMT sought to rehabilitate heavy heroin users by using methadone to block the "euphorigenic potential of heroin" (Pearson 1970, 2571). By blocking the temptation for heroin, MMT interrupts the cycle of craving, tolerance, and antisocial behavior (Kleber and Kellerman 1971, 380). MMT was akin to the lifetime treatment of diabetics using insulin; MMT had a low cost and could reduce both hepatitis C transmission and property crimes (Kleinman 1977, 208; Methadone Maintenance 1969, 1176).

Studies reported that after five months of treatment 45 percent of people had an increase in employment, with increases to 61 percent after 11 months and 85 percent after 12 months (Methadone Maintenance 1969, 1178). Detoxification clinics having no clinical services (e.g., individual or group counseling) only separated the patient from heroin for a short period of time when compared to institutions with more intensive treatment practices (Methadone Maintenance 1969, 1179). Yet Barbara Pearson argued as early as 1970 that "only pennies a day are needed for freedom of the shackles of heroin addiction," so some organizations provided only detoxification without incorporating behavioral therapy (Pearson 1970, 2571). Detoxification was necessary (usually lasting no longer than four to seven days of treatment), but clients without continued treatment were likely to relapse.

In 1998, the General Accounting Office (now Government Accountability Office) noted that large-scale studies show that substance abusers offered extended harm-reduction treatment were less likely to take part in criminal activity (General Accounting Office 1998, 3). ONDCP also stated that "studies and statistics indicate that the fastest and most cost effective way to reduce the demand for illicit drugs is to treat chronic hard core drug users" (ONDCP 1995). Some estimates suggest that a dollar invested in drug treatment saved $7.46 in societal costs; by contrast, taxpayers lose almost 80 cents for every dollar spent on enforcement-based policy (Rydell and Everingham 1994).

Presidential Attention to Treatment and Heroin

As documented in the case of MMT, only the Nixon administration truly advocated harm-reduction drug policies. Presidents before and after Nixon handled the drug problem with law enforcement. The metaphor of the "War on Drugs" reinforces the role of such efforts to stop the flow and use of drugs. A 1995 Chicago Council on Foreign Relations national survey showed that 85 percent of people supported military power on foreign soil to seize drugs, with equal support from both Republicans and Democrats (Falco 1996, 120). Little attention was paid to the relative efficacy of treatment.

Metaphors in policymaking are powerful tools for gaining support. Metaphors crafted by policymakers and members of society can help simplify complicated issues conceptually. Politicians can use well-chosen metaphors to support an agenda and help move it to the forefront of the public (or institutional) agenda. Metaphors help people operate in ambiguous contexts (Lakoff and Johnson 1980; Morone 2003; Whitford and Yates 2009). The central idea here is that metaphors simplify and structure the choices that decision makers face (e.g., "just say no" in the case of the War on Drugs).

According to Lakoff and Johnson (1980), metaphor helps people function in everyday contexts. Metaphor is systematic and orientational. A useful example in their exposition is the metaphor "argument is war." Because metaphor is both systematic and orientational, whole hosts of affiliated concepts accompany the overall governing metaphor of "argument is war." For example, we experience and use the supporting metaphors of "win," "loss," "opponent," "attack," "defend," "gain," "plan," "strategies," and "defensible." The structure of war becomes affiliated with the structure of argument, so the metaphor itself systematizes and orients the actions we experience and perform in the process of arguing.

Likewise, the War on Drugs is a prominent example of the use of a "war metaphor," a tactic used in many other policy arenas, such as the war on terrorism or poverty. Using the term "war" as a metaphor in policymaking is a powerful way to shape public impressions of the dangers inherent in public issues, and is a tool for gaining the support of those who need convincing during the policy process, particularly in societies that favor war or the use of power to solve problems (Campbell 2002, 32). The metaphor War on Drugs has helped maintain narcotics-control policy for the past 20 years. It has helped create both policies that have been deemed "successes" and others that appear unsuccessful. Both types have proven difficult to remove because they were created using the rhetoric of war (Campbell 2002, 28-29). Once these programs are established, politicians often back them because they are familiar. That familiarity makes players unlikely to risk their political careers by expressing or pursuing new or extreme ideas (Campbell 2002, 29). Those metaphors systematize and orient the actions of many types of actors involved in the policy process, just as politicians and policymakers have found themselves engaged in a War on Drugs. Citizens also find their actions systematized and oriented by the war metaphor.

Programmatic ideas are specific kinds of metaphors that describe ways to create and implement policies that can be used across policy domains (e.g., "cost-benefit analysis"). Programmatic ideas are especially useful for actors looking to build quick coalitions because they are expressed in the "simplest and strongest" terms (Campbell 2002, 29). A consequence has been that high-budget drug policies continue to receive funding. We discuss below the specific way that enforcement and treatment are the key programmatic ideas that shape the behavior of participants in the policy process defining narcotics-control policy.

When practicing their extra-constitutional role as chief legislator, presidents often rely on the use of metaphors and the programmatic ideas that support them. Setting the public agenda is crucial because of the president's considerable potential influence on the formulation of public policies. In practice, legislators have too little time and resources to make well-formed policy. New ideas—even those introduced by presidents—face fierce competition and examination. Presidents who want to shift the debate closer to their preferred outcome use metaphors to spur interest, but they must also couple those metaphors with programmatic ideas if they want them to find a place on the agenda (Anderson 2000, 88). The debate the presidents seek to control, then, is the debate between conflicting perceptions of a problem. Politicians will resolve those perceptions, and how they do so will determine the kinds of policy solutions they devise. Presidents have power. They influence people, and they rely on rhetoric and metaphor to do so.

Political scientists have long debated the president's role in using rhetoric to shape the flow of power and influence in the American policy process. Two classic studies saw the president's role in terms of guide and teacher. Rossiter (1960) saw the president as an American "moral spokesman," while Neustadt (1960, 9) saw rhetoric as the president's way of serving as a "teacher to the public" (100-107). More advanced studies describe the president's rhetorical role as bridging "two constitutions" (Tulis 1987). The "first constitution" pinned the executive in a system of checks and balances. The "second constitution" developed in the twentieth century when presidents sought to move around Congress and the Court's checks and balances by speaking directly to the people through appeals. Probably the most synthetic view comes from Kernell (1997), who suggests that the president "goes public" to change how the democracy deliberates over public policy. Data show how presidential addresses, appearances, and travel change over time. Trends change along with innovations in radio, television, and the Internet. Ronald Reagan and Harry Truman, along with others, used appeals as a core policy strategy.

No studies have documented exactly how and when presidents stopped talking about substance-abuse treatment options for solving the problem of drug abuse. Our data for this section of the paper come from the American Presidency Project, located at the University of California, Santa Barbara (UCSB), which contains records of all public papers of the President of the United States.[4] This is the only online resource to have consolidated, coded, and organized into a single searchable database the messages and papers of Presidents Washington through Taft (covering 1789 to 1913), the public papers of Presidents Hoover through Bush (from 1929 to 1993), and presidential documents from Presidents Clinton and G.W. Bush (covering 1993 to 2007). John Woolley and Gerhard Peters of UCSB made the data available for public use in 1999.

We used four different combinations of terms to search the database for speeches that the presidents gave between January 1, 1789, and December 31, 2007. These searches helped identify the documents that represent our sample for the study. The content analysis of the documents consisted of searches using the following term(s): "harm reduction," "methadone," "heroin and treatment," and "war on drugs." We selected these specifically due to their use in the literature review and because they are terms often used by presidents when describing drug policy. We want to describe how presidential statements changed over a long time period. We focus on the time period from 1962 to 2007.

We believe these are useful search terms in the context of discussions about dealing with "the drug problem" from a treatment perspective. We show below how other measures capture other elements of narcotics-control policy.

---

[4] Frontline, "Frontline: Drug Wars."

We begin by noting that when speaking about these issues, presidents most likely used the terms "heroin" and "treatment." Specifically, there are no records of a president ever using the term "harm reduction" in a public statement. Moreover, the use of the term "methadone" has only been recorded seven times—and most of these occurred during Nixon's years in office.

We note that presidents used the term "War on Drugs" only five more times than "heroin" and "treatment"—and when we examined the contents of those documents it was clear that they included many topics besides narcotics policy. Here, we focus on the records associated with heroin and treatment and not the War on Drugs. Specifically, we use the search term "heroin and treatment" to measure when the president's public agenda addressed the element of treatment in the context of narcotics-control policy. In contrast to a more general discussion of narcotics, we believe that presidents who spoke more about heroin and treatment during a term signaled a stronger orientation toward treatment (e.g., see Whitford and Yates 2009).

Figure 1. Number of Mentions of Heroin and Treatment, 1962–2007

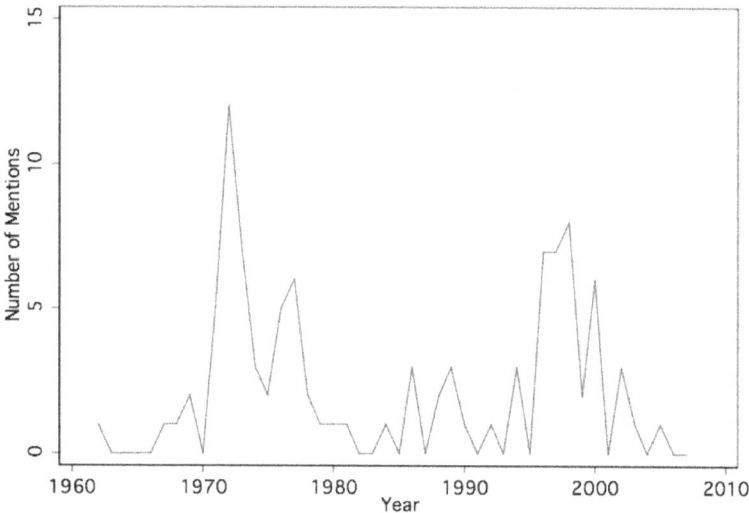

Data Source: The American Presidency Project. n.d. http://www.presidency.uscb.

Our data include the 45 years since 1962 in which a president mentioned heroin treatment in a documented report. Figure 1 shows how mentions of heroin and treatment have ebbed and flowed over time. The first peak is in 1972 in the Nixon administration, while the second, smaller peak is in 1998 in the Clinton administration. There are deep "troughs" of inattention—especially during the Reagan and George H.W. Bush administrations, which were also the peak of the War on Drugs metaphor.

Table 1 shows the total attention paid by each presidential administration to treatment options for heroin abusers, as recorded in the public papers of the president. Total attention means the number of times a president is on record for using the terms "heroin" and "treatment" in the same message. The two peaks again are the Nixon and Clinton administrations, although this portrait reveals that the total attention paid by the Clinton administration was greater than that during the Nixon administration (although, of course, Clinton actually served longer in office). There was virtually no attention paid to these options before Nixon. The three most recent Republican administrations have paid only minuscule attention—a total of 17 mentions over a 19-year time period.

Table 1: Presidential Agendas Regarding Drug Treatment for Heroin

President	Number of mentions
Kennedy	1
Johnson	2
Nixon	29
Ford	7
Carter	10
Reagan	7
Bush, G.H.W.	5
Clinton	33
Bush, G.W.	5

Data Source: The American Presidency Project. n.d. http://www.presidency.uscb.

Surprisingly, as Table 2 shows, Republican presidents in total were more likely to discuss heroin and the treatment option than were Democrats: 53.5 percent of mentions occurred during a Republican administration. However, the data also show that Republican attention was largely a 1970s-era phenomenon. Specifically, when Nixon's attention is subtracted from the Republican numbers, there were only 24 mentions of heroin and treatment by Republicans. Of course, when Clinton is subtracted from the Democrat total, there were only 13, but then 3 of those 13 mentions predate the heroin surge experienced during the Nixon administration.

Table 2. Drug Policy Agenda-Setting by Political Party

Party of president	Frequency of mentions	Percentage of total mentions
Republican	53	53.5
Democrat	46	46.5
Total	99	100.0

Data Source: The American Presidency Project. n.d. http://www.presidency.uscb.

In total, the attention spike starting in the late 1960s and early 1970s was followed by a sharp decline in the president's mentions of drug treatment during the 1970s. The data do not reveal a significant increase until the mid-1990s to the beginning of 2000. These trends describe neither the total War on Drugs nor the funding spent on drug programs, which explains the low frequency in the 1980s when the drug war was at its highest point during Reagan's tenure.

The data on drug trends among U.S. citizens display peaks during similar time periods (ONDCP 2002). The height of drug use was 1979, just after the Nixon administration emphasized drug treatment. By 1985, drug use began to fall, until it recorded its lowest reported use in 1992. Drug treatment policy also cycled off the presidents' agendas. By 1994 to 1998, the United States saw increased drug use.

We contrast the data presented above with data on the reported use of marijuana, which as we noted above was strongly considered for decriminalization during the 1970s.[5] Our data come from the National Household Survey on Drug Abuse (NHSDA) and the Substance Abuse and Mental

---

[5] We do not offer a full statistical model of these processes for the reason that our time periods are significantly shorter and our data substantially coarser than we would need in order to apply an advanced time series approach such as generalized autoregressive conditional heteroskedasticity (GARCH) models; nor do our data have qualities necessary for the estimation of Granger causality through the use of vector autoregression (VAR) models. Instead, we rely here on graphical analysis and interpretation to extend our point about how treatment was not part of the larger enforcement-oriented narcotics control regime.

Health Services Administration (SAMHSA). Figure 2 shows the incidence of daily marijuana use among 12th-grade high school students. There was reported heavy marijuana usage just prior to Reagan's first term, but usage dropped throughout the 1980s until the beginning of the Clinton administration. It is argued that these data on narcotics use (at least marijuana) for this age cohort shaped the beginning of the enforcement-based War on Drugs of the Reagan administration (Whitford and Yates 2009).

Figure 3 shows estimates of new drug use initiation, by type of drug, from data gathered from the National Household Survey on Drug Abuse conducted by the National Institute on Drug Abuse (NIDA). The most remarkable aspect of this for our claim here is that heroin initiation is relatively flat throughout the series.

Figure 2. Percentage of 12th Graders Who Use Marijuana on a Daily Basis, 1975–2005

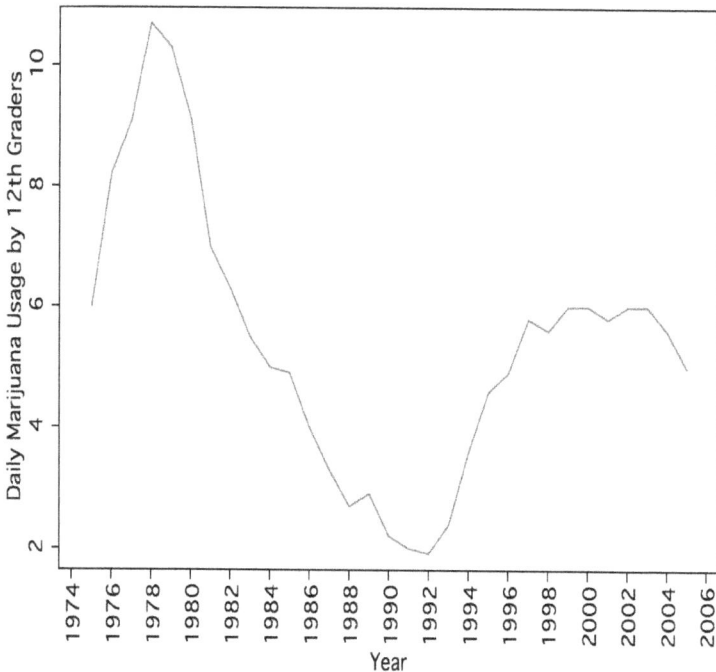

Data Source: National Household Survey on Drug Abuse (NHSDA), conducted by the National Institute of Drug Abuse (NIDA); and the Substance Abuse and Mental Health Services Administration (SAMHSA).

Figure 3. New Initiates (in thousands) of Marijuana, Cocaine, Hallucinogens, and Heroin, 1962–1990

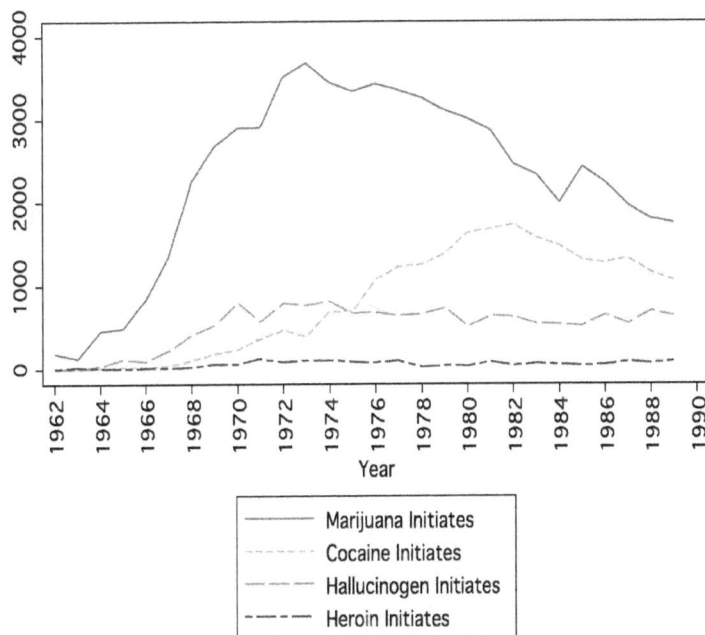

Data Source: National Household Survey on Drug Abuse (NHSDA), conducted by the National Institute on Drug Abuse (NIDA)

Perhaps the best evidence of the implementation of the War on Drugs by the federal government is incarceration of individuals for federal drug crimes. Figure 4 shows how this changed over the 1970–1998 time period. Our data come from the Sourcebook of Criminal Justice Statistics 2000, produced by the Bureau of Justice Statistics. Drug offenders constituted less than 25 percent of federal prison inmates in 1980; that figure was over 60 percent by 1994. Clearly, the War on Drugs has changed the composition of the federal prison population.

Figure 4. Percentage of the Federal Prison Population Incarcerated for Drug Offenses, 1970–1998

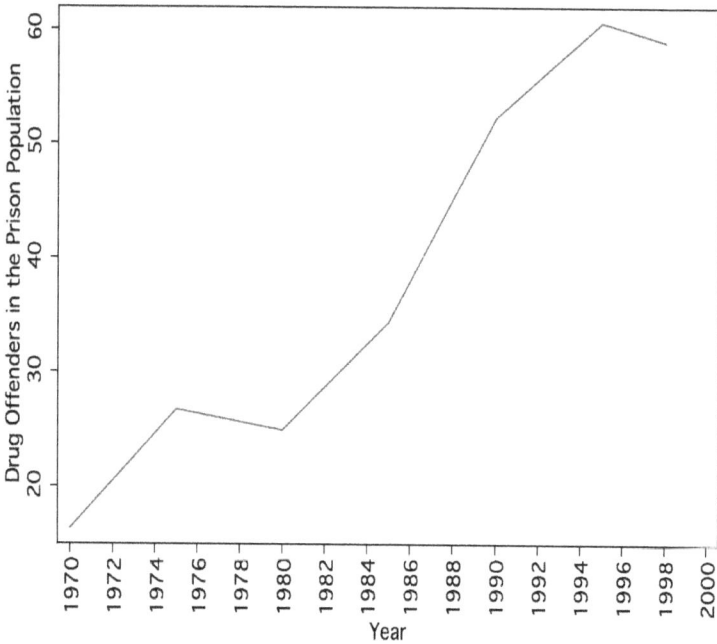

Data Source: Sourcebook of Criminal Justice Statistics 2000 (Bureau of Justice Statistics).

      Drug policy rose to a higher level on the presidential agenda in the 1960s, when Nixon created agencies and increased federal spending for solving the drug problem. Drug use during this period was at its highest recorded level in U.S. history up to this point, so government prioritized education and treatment. After the 1970s, drug use decreased in the population even after the introduction of crack cocaine in the 1980s. Heroin after this time saw limited—although persistent—use. Yet as discussed above, the 1980s' "supply side" approach to enforcement has limitations, one of which has been the change in the street price of illicit drugs. The data we offer here show that treatment is a priority only when drug use is on the rise. Of course, agencies with missions and goals related to the illicit use of drugs also manipulate perceptions that are based on policy metaphors. Enforcement budgets often fall when drug use declines; rhetoric may be a strategy for avoiding that outcome (Epstein 1990, 36). But when drug use increases, the money required for treatment is lower and the impact is clearer in terms of reducing use—so the president responds accordingly.

      As Tulis notes, the president's ability to lead the agenda is extra-constitutional—that is, it exists only in the sense that the president can and chooses to dominate the market of ideas. The president competes with other groups seeking to control that agenda—some of which have more reason to stay actively involved in the debate over the mechanisms of power and policy. One reason for this attempt to counterbalance the president is because of these swings of attention and inattention that are probably tracking changes in the preferences of the larger population.

Discussion

Presidents have used the bully pulpit to create rhetoric for the War on Drugs that has, in turn, produced a criminal justice system overwhelmed with drug-related crimes. In contrast, scientific evidence supports the use of methadone maintenance for the treatment of heroin addiction. We argue that the agenda has shifted away from treatment options for heroin. This shift has happened when there has been increased use of drugs.

In contrast, hardcore heroin users could and do benefit from this harm-reduction strategy—even though presidents presiding over the War on Drugs have largely ignored it. This has left the job of shifting the rhetorical agenda to interests outside the political process who have a continuing interest in these special populations. Nonprofit organizations that emphasize drug treatment may act as a counterbalance to a political system in which presidents pay important but largely transitory attention to the problem of opiate addiction and other long-term drug problems. The reason for this need for a counterbalance is quite simple: presidents (and the agencies who serve them and implement the law) construct rhetorical agendas—populated by policy metaphors and building on programmatic ideas—with their own interests in mind. In the War on Drugs, the past 30 years have seen an elevation of enforcement efforts and less emphasis on cost-effective substance-abuse treatment.

We recognize that there are limitations to the arguments we have presented here. We do not describe in great detail how the scientific community has changed its own perceptions of treatment. Neither do we describe shifting patterns of support among the public for treatment options. One reason for this is that we do not have systematic data on public opinion regarding treatment options; in fact, systematic data on public opinion regarding the "drug problem" are very coarse, to the degree that we cannot readily distinguish exactly what the public cares about in this arena (e.g., marijuana, heroin, cocaine, and methamphetamines). Likewise, we do not describe to a great degree what the presidents have understood about drugs—just their degree of attention. This is common in the policy agendas literature, and is a useful complaint about many studies. We believe our paper gives reason for future studies to investigate exactly what the president means when he talks about drugs, particularly given the range of individual experiences that presidents acknowledge in their own lives (e.g., Ford's understanding of treatment, other presidents' actual usage experiences). Finally, an important missing element is a full understanding of the extent to which nonprofit and other nongovernmental organizations have influenced the debate on dealing with drugs toward treatment rather than incarceration. We would benefit from knowing whether such organizations have tried to be heard (and their use of resources in doing so), and similarly why their effects have been so small.

Conclusions

We close by noting four themes that warrant special emphasis for building a full understanding of the president's role in shaping narcotics-control policy, especially with regard to treatment options. First, the evidence is clear in other cases that general presidential attention to narcotics—and not just treatment—has an impact on the federal government's implementation of the War on Drugs. Whitford and Yates (2009) show sizeable shifts in enforcement following presidential attention. Second, we again emphasize our claim that enforcement has replaced treatment—as evidenced in the data on enforcement and incarceration. While demand reduction is a valuable approach to reducing the presence of drugs in society, most strategies center on supply reduction. Our partial explanation is that presidents shaped this process by deemphasizing treatment options, especially in the case of heroin use. Third, we note that other studies, such as Morone (2003), show how pervasive this dynamic is in American politics. In a wide array of experiences, mostly involving issues core to "morality policy," American policy tends to overweight punishment and underweight rehabilitation. The metaphor of war comes into play again and again. It is systematic and it orients policy debates and public opinion by shaping who we consider "innocent" and worthy of protection and who we consider "decadent" and worthy of punishment (e.g., users). Fourth, our paper does not address current and important laws that work to support treatment strategies, such as the Drug Addiction Treatment Act of 2000 (Substance Abuse and Mental Health Services Administration 2000). This Act seeks to improve the regulation of MMT by focusing on how providers implement treatment strategies, but also by trying to build a knowledge base to improve those approaches (Marion 2005). A full treatment of those developments is beyond the scope of this paper, but understanding why and how President Clinton contributed to that act is useful for understanding recent developments in how presidents address treatment for heroin addiction.

The president's powers are servants to his political interests. In the long run, solutions for America's heroin problem flow from the tension between these competing interests. While the peaks and valleys of presidential attention may occasionally find heroin worth talking about, the long-term problem of abuse can be solved only when organizations with particularistic concerns are also able to shape the policy agenda.

References

Anderson, J.E. 2000. *Public Policymaking: An Introduction*. Boston: Houghton Mifflin.

Austin, J., and J. Irwin. 2001. *It's About Time: America's Imprisonment Binge*, Fifth Edition. Belmont, CA: Wadsworth.

Belenko, S.R. 2001. *Drugs and Drug Policy in America: A Documented History*. Westport, CT: Greenwood Press.

Brecher, E.M. 1972. *Licit and Illicit Drugs*. Little, Brown.

Campbell, J.L. 2002. "Ideas, Politics, and Public Policy." *Annual Review of Sociology* 28: 28-32.

Conser, J.A., G.D. Russell, R. Paynich, and T.E. Gingerich. 2001. *Law Enforcement in the United States*. New York: Aspen Publishers.

DuPont, R.L., and M.H. Greene. 1973. "The Dynamics of the Heroin Addiction Epidemic." *Science* 181: 716-721.

Epstein, E.J. 1990. *Agency of Fear: Opiates and Political Power in America*. London: Verso.

Falco, Mathea. 1996. "U.S. Drug Policy: Addicted to Failure." *Foreign Policy* 102: 120-121.

General Accounting Office. 1998. *Drug Abuse: Studies Show Treatment Is Effective, But Benefits May Be Overstated*. GAO/HEHS-98-72.

Goode, Erich. 1997. *Between Politics and Reason: The Drug Legalization Debate*. New York: St. Martin's Press.

Holder, H.D. 1998. "Cost Benefits of Substance Abuse Treatment: An Overview of Results from Alcohol and Drug Abuse." *Journal of Mental Health Policy and Economics* 1 (1): 23-29.

Kernell, Samuel. 1997. *Going Public: New Strategies of Presidential Leadership*, Third Edition. Washington, DC: CQ Press.

Kleber, H., and G.L. Kellerman. 1971. "Current Issues in Methadone Treatment of Heroin Dependence." *Medical Care* 9: 379-80.

Kleinman, P.H. 1977. "The Magic Fix: A Critical Analysis of Methadone Maintenance Treatment." *Social Problems* 25 (2): 208-214.

Lakoff, G., and M. Johnson. 1980. *Metaphors We Live By*. Chicago: University of Chicago Press.

Levine, D., P. Stoloff, and N. Spruill. 1976. "Public Drug Treatment and Addict Crime." *The Journal of Legal Studies* 5: 435-439.

Marion, I.J. 2005. "Methadone Treatment at Forty." *NIDA Science & Practice Perspectives* 3 (1): 25-31.

Massing, M. 1998. *The Fix*. New York: Simon & Schuster.

"Methadone." 1948. *Life Magazine*, 90. New York.

Morone, J. 2003. *Hellfire Nation: The Politics of Sin in American History*. New Haven, CT: Yale University Press.

Musto, D. 1987. *The American Disease: Origins of Narcotic Control*. Oxford: Oxford University Press.

Neustadt, R.E. 1960. *Presidential Power: The Politics of Leadership*. New York: John Wiley & Sons.

Office of National Drug Control Policy (ONDCP). 1995. *National Drug Control Policy Strategy Report*.

Office of National Drug Control Policy (ONDCP). 2002. "Drug Use Trends." October. http://www.whitehousedrugpolicy.gov/publications/factsht/druguse/.

Parenti, C. 2000. *Lockdown America: Police and Prisons in the Age of Crisis*, New Edition. London: Verso.

Pearson, B.A. 1970. "The Program at Beth Israel Medical Center." *American Journal of Nursing* 70: 2571.

Preston, Andrew and Gerald Bennett. 2003. "The History of Methadone and Methadone Prescribing." In *Methadone Matters: Evolving Community Treatment of Opiate Addiction*, eds. Gillian Tober and John Strang. London: Taylor and Francis, 13.

Rossiter, C. 1960. *The American Presidency*. New York: Harcourt Brace.

Rydell, C.P., and S.S. Everingham. 1994. *Controlling Cocaine XVI*. Drug Policy Research Center, RAND Corporation, for Office of National Drug Control Policy and the United States Army.

Schleif, W. 1901. "New Drugs." *American Journal of Nursing* 1: 429.

Substance Abuse and Mental Health Services Administration (SAMHSA). 2000. *Drug Addiction Treatment Act of 2000*. Rockville, MD: SAMHSA. http://buprenorphine.samhsa.gov/data.html.

Tulis, Jeffrey K. 1987. *The Rhetorical Presidency*. Princeton, NJ: Princeton University Press.

Whitford, A., and J. Yates. 2003. "Policy Signals and Executive Governance: Presidential Rhetoric in the War on Drugs." *Journal of Politics* 65 (4): 995-1012.

Whitford, A., and J. Yates. 2009. *Presidential Rhetoric and the Public Agenda: Constructing the War on Drugs*. Baltimore, MD: The Johns Hopkins University Press.

Wright, P. 2003. *Prison Nation: The Warehousing of America's Poor*. New York: Routledge.

U.S. Tobacco Control: Six Lessons in Public Policy for Medical and Science Professionals

Catherine E. Rudder, *George Mason University*
A. Lee Fritschler, *George Mason University*

Introduction

As early as the 1890s, the scientific community suspected that cigarette smoking in particular and tobacco use in general was a threat to health. By the 1950s, the body of evidence-based science grew to a stronger and more convincing body of published research. Yet, such findings were largely ignored by the general public who were bombarded with advertising promoting the glamour of smoking and by their governments. In the mid-1960s, actions taken by individuals in the scientific and political communities moved tobacco control to the public agenda in ways which made it possible for incremental but significant policy changes to be made over the next 45 years.

Once smoking was officially recognized as harmful, it took decades for political support for regulation of tobacco to approach a majority in Congress. Over the years a health coalition grew and gained sufficient power to engage policymaking mechanisms to create tobacco control policies. Near herculean political effort over a protracted period was required fully to match the entrenched power of tobacco interests. Health professionals were committed to the struggle, and without them the chances are good that new policy directions would not have been adopted. [1]

Why was there such fierce resistance to change in policy that would promote public health? Even when hundreds of thousands of deaths in the United States each year were traced to tobacco-related causes—ranging from lung and laryngeal cancers to chronic pulmonary obstructive heart and ischemic heart disease—the public seemed willing to ignore the data and leave the policy arena under the control of pro-tobacco forces. [2] This article explores some of the reasons for political inertia and active resistance to regulation of tobacco, and some of the methods that were used to surmount them. Methods that have reduced the prevalence of smoking are being applied by health professionals to attack the problem of obesity (Engelhard, Garson, and Dorn 2009). Similarly, *political* techniques that have been employed to fight pro-tobacco forces can be applied to a wide variety of policy controversies of concern to the scientific and medical communities.

The number of tobacco-related deaths remains staggering although the percentage of smokers in the population has declined dramatically. According to the Centers for Disease Control and Prevention (2006), smoking declined by 20 percent over the period 1997–2007, a decline which

---

[1] Those new directions included a range of policy approaches including health warning labels on cigarette packages and in advertising, limits on advertising, smoking bans in public places, liability determinations, support for new medical devices, public education and punitive excises, and sales taxes on cigarettes. Studies show that higher cigarette taxes are one of the most effective ways to reduce smoking among both youth and adults. Every 10 percent increase in the price of cigarettes reduces youth smoking by about seven percent and overall cigarette consumption by about four percent (Higher Cigarette Taxes: Reducing Smoking Saves Lives Saves Money, July 31, 2009, http://www.tobaccofreekids.org/ reports/prices/). Also particularly effective was equal-time advertising that allowed public health advocates to broadcast one anti-smoking advertisement for every two placed by cigarette companies.

[2] By 1964 the connection between smoking, on the one hand, and lung and laryngeal cancer, on the other, in men was clearly established on the basis of 7,000 articles in the biomedical literature (Centers for Disease Control and Prevention).

coincided with implementation of the 1998 tobacco out-of-court settlement between the states of the Union and the major tobacco companies. Although 20 percent of American adults—disproportionately low income and people of color—smoke, halving of the proportion of smokers as well as large decline in new users are signal victories for health proponents.[3]

Drawing from the example of the battle over use of tobacco in the United States, this article identifies six political lessons for science professionals desirous of effectively using scientific research to inform public policy in democratic societies. These lessons are derived from the culture of politics where policy development is not linear but highly contingent, often unpredictable, and dependent on convincing people to recognize the existence of a problem and the best way to resolve it. Outcomes result from building majorities, not from scientific expertise. Nevertheless, such expertise needs to be integrated, even if imperfectly, into policy. Tobacco politics in the United States demonstrates that good science can influence policy outcomes, but the way requires persistence, strategic action, and understanding of the political territory, as the lessons below demonstrate.

Lesson 1: Make the message simple and clear

Some issues in health and medical policy are handled in the political arena more easily and with more dispatch than others. Two particularly important variables which separate the easier from more difficult issues are the (1) degree of the complexity of scientific findings adduced to support a policy shift and (2) the degree to which interests that clash with the proposed shift are politically organized and embedded in society. As Figure 1 illustrates, the optimal position (a pattern of weak interests and simple science) is in the top left-hand corner, indicated by the arrows.

Figure 1: Politics of Public Policy Impelled by Technical or Scientific Understanding

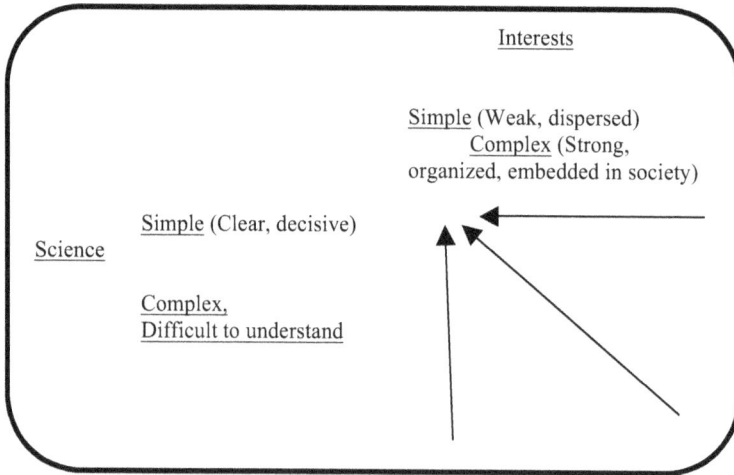

By its nature the scientific enterprise is premised upon lack of certainty. Nevertheless, *ceteris paribus*, the more decisive the findings and the more clearly communicated their implications for people's lives, the more likely that science will be taken into account in policymaking. At the same time, to the degree that the prosperity of existing interests are threatened by a policy shift, even relatively decisive, clear results of research may be insufficient to motivate a policy change.

---

[3] Twenty percent constitutes 45 million adults, with 438,000 people each year dying prematurely from smoking-related causes. Since the seminal surgeon general's report of 1964 (see below), perhaps 15 million Americans have died from smoking-related causes.

112

Multiple, well-financed and politically organized interests can stop progressive change in its tracks. This combination of strong interests and complex science helps explain the cold reception that findings, for example, on global warming initially received in the halls of governance.[4]

In the case of tobacco control, clear and decisive findings that smoking leads to numerous chronic and fatal diseases piled up over the years (Centers for Disease Control and Prevention 2004). The dissemination of scientific studies in popular outlets gradually made denial of smoking's harms virtually impossible. Still, tobacco companies continued to argue that the evidence was not yet conclusive, allowing diehards to lie to themselves that using tobacco was okay. As the science became increasingly decisive and clearly communicated, the entrenched tobacco interests remained implacable with the result that even after the medical science was clear the national policy environment did not give way to regulation. Pro-tobacco forces continued to dominate Congress throughout the twentieth century and to do the bidding of the tobacco industry.

Lesson 2: Many important matters affecting the public never reach the agenda of policymakers

The most effective way to deal with a matter that disrupts the status quo is simply to be sure it stays off the agendas of those policymakers who could alter it (Bachrach and Baratz 1962). That is exactly the strategy that the pro-tobacco forces followed. In 1906, with the passage of the first Food and Drug Act, nicotine, the active ingredient in tobacco, was officially excluded as a designated "drug" or as a proper subject for regulation by any federal agency. Through most of the century these actions effectively kept tobacco control advocates on the sidelines and their issue off the national agenda.

The situation was radically changed in 1964 when one courageous public official decided to act unilaterally. At that time the Surgeon General of the United States, Dr. Luther Terry—a physician and otherwise relatively politically powerless appointee of the president—single-handedly moved the issue of smoking to the national agenda. He used his position as chief medical officer of the United States to issue an authoritative report declaring smoking to be a health hazard. The issue of smoking and health arose in a 1962 nationally televised press conference of President Kennedy. A member of the press corps asked what the president planned to do to address the issue. Caught off-guard, the president said he would respond in a week and then asked the Public Health Service to report what it had been doing on the smoking question. That impromptu response, to the chagrin of tobacco interests and the relief of many concerned about public health, placed the smoking issue on the national agenda, however, tentatively. Within two weeks Dr. Terry announced that he would form an advisory committee to study the matter. This series of events led to the ground-breaking 1964 Surgeon General's Report (Department of Health, Education, and Welfare 1964). True, Congress had no intention of legislating any changes, but another method to begin to change policy—through one of the administrative agencies—would be found and would force Congress to respond in order to prevent the establishment of new policy too inimical to tobacco interests.

Anti-smoking activists took advantage of the opening provided by the president. Policy entrepreneurs and some courageous leaders in government created novel arguments and publicized the latest findings of medical researchers to keep the issue alive. Helping keep tobacco control on the agendas of policymakers over time, subsequent surgeons-general issued reports on the damage caused by cigarettes and other tobacco products. The Centers for Disease Control and Prevention (CDC) contributed to publicizing the harms of smoking to the voting public, as did anti-smoking organizations which also lobbied governmental bodies to regulate tobacco use.

---

[4] A particularly useful source to consult concerning the use of expertise in the policy process is Giandomenico Majone's *Evidence, Policy and Persuasion in the Policy Process* (Majone 1992).

Lesson 3:   To succeed in policy change and innovation, control the definition of the issue

Political scientist E. E. Schattschneider's (1960) classic work on political strategy, *The Semisovereign People,* argues that "the definition of the alternatives is the *supreme instrument* of power" [emphasis his]. The idea here is for proponents to define or frame an issue so that, in effect, they win. The issue is articulated in such a way that one's opponents are forced into the minority position and that the desired outcome becomes the majority position. Of course, opponents are simultaneously trying to frame the issue to *their* advantage. Whichever side's definition of the issue predominates is the side that succeeds.

Until the 1960s tobacco was seen, or framed, primarily as an agricultural and financial matter. Many farmers, backed up by powerful members of Congress from five or six Southern conservative, tobacco-growing states, responded vigorously and negatively to any attempt to initiate controls on tobacco consumption. Tobacco and its related industries formed the financial backbone of those states, they argued. In fact, the number of people dependent on tobacco for their livelihood constituted a substantial portion of the working population of those states. Farmers, their suppliers, tobacco product manufacturers and state officials dependent upon tobacco tax revenues were adamant about preserving the status quo. Tobacco supporters had strong allies around the country including advertising agencies, magazines, and newspapers that relied on revenues from cigarette advertising and retailers selling tobacco products.

As tobacco control became a more salient issue, smokers, too, became more vocal and generally sided with the pro-tobacco forces. Consistent with the American culture of individualism, to many smokers the matter was one of free choice. Reinforced by tobacco companies' arguments, people with a libertarian bent, whether smokers or not, abhorred paternalistic government dictating individual behavior. The multiple frames of economic survival and free choice worked in conjunction with tobacco companies efforts to align as many interests as possible on their side. The companies generously helped fund symphony orchestras, nonprofit minority and women's groups, museums and other cultural activities. Tobacco philanthropy had the efficacious effect of neutralizing opposition from the upper middle class patrons of cultural institutions, and of creating support from groups, like African-Americans, who were targeted by the companies for increased rates of tobacco consumption.

The scientific findings whose implications were that smoking causes chronic health problems and premature death were attacked frontally. The frame here was to shift attention from science and probabilities to absolute certainty. Correlation (no matter how high) is not equivalent to causation, said pro-tobacco forces. For example, smokers were found to have much higher rates of heart failure. The pro-tobacco forces asserted that medical researchers could not *prove* that smoking causes heart disease; maybe so-called Type A personalities were more likely to smoke, suggesting a spurious connection between smoking and death.

More alarmingly for the scientific community, the tobacco companies managed to co-opt leading researchers at institutions like Harvard University to perform research that helped slow the movement toward government regulation of smoking (Frontline 1998). Here, then, the frame was "the jury is out"; "we don't know enough yet to regulate"; "we are waiting for more findings"; "not even the best researchers in the country are certain." As shown in Figure 1, the companies were successfully moving the science toward complexity and had increased the number of people with an interest in tobacco's success.

Many members of Congress adopted and used these multiple issue frames in order to defeat anti-tobacco, public health advocates who were greatly out-numbered, out-organized, and poorly financed. Tobacco interests were concentrated, and public health proponents (including families who had lost loved ones in agonizing deaths from the effects of smoking) were dispersed. This array of concentrated versus dispersed interests almost always guarantees a favorable outcome for the former (Olson 1965).

114

Though Congress was controlled by conservative, Southern senators and representatives who were pro-tobacco, a few individual members of Congress heroically worked to alter the political equation and to provide a single alternative frame: The issue of smoking is a matter of public health, of life and death, and, hence a *public* policy issue that must be addressed by government. Attempts like these to change the cultural/ agricultural/financial/scientific issue frames failed to budge the congressional supporters of the tobacco industry. A way had to be found to move the issue to another policy venue and to take control of issue framing out of the hands of the tobacco companies (Kingdon 2002).

One stunning example of innovative framing emanated from new scientific research that pointed to passive smoking (the inhalation of smoke, called second-hand smoke, SHS, or environmental tobacco smoke, ETS) as the culprit in many illnesses of non-smokers who had been persistently exposed to smokers' exhaust fumes (National Research Council 1986). This research, which was replicated and tightened over time, became increasingly difficult to ignore, despite tobacco companies' barrage of counter-arguments and seeming obfuscation. Now the deleterious impact of smoking could be seen not as the result of a personal choice (and hence no one else's business), but as harming innocent people, including children and workers forced to inhale others' smoke in the course of their employment. Even in America's individualistic culture, regulation of cigarettes found a clear moral justification, thanks to scientific research publicized and made understandable to the general public. Even though Congress remained hostile to the regulation of smoking, state and local governments and federal agencies began to limit—and eventually outlaw—smoking in buildings and other enclosed spaces like aircrafts.

Lesson 4: If the way is blocked, change venues, or "Life is simpler when you plow around the stump" (Anonymous)

Too often people tend to think of government as a single institution. This notion is in error, as there are in effect many governments—that is, governmental arenas beyond the national legislature—where policy is made within democratic nations. Furthermore, international organizations like the World Health Organization (WHO) that are making public policy have opened another set of venues for change (Rudder 2008).

The opportunities created by multiple points of access are especially abundant in federal systems like that of the United States The American system, characterized by substantial policy power vested in the states, multiplies the number of venues that can be employed to effect policy change. As the European Union strengthens its own institutions, it too is creating alternative venues to the single state system that has dominated Europe for centuries.

Beyond federalism as a venue-creating institution, the reality of multiple points of access is reflected in the fact that within modern government much policymaking authority has been delegated to administrative agencies. In many nations such bodies have the authority to write rules and regulations that have the same enforcement effects as law passed by a legislature. A combination of shifting the venue and creating an issue frame to fit the venue can be a winning strategy.

In the tobacco control case, Congress's initial refusal to act in the 1960s led to the search for another policy lever. Proponents for regulating tobacco experienced their first success when they managed to wrest the issue away from its old venues, Congress and the Department of Agriculture, and transfer it to a new one, the Federal Trade Commission (FTC)—a designated "independent agency" of the federal government—which was much more sympathetic to health consequences than either Congress or Agriculture was at the time. Michael Pertshuk, who later became Chairman of the FTC, devised a way to frame the issue of smoking that placed the matter squarely in the jurisdiction of his agency. Tobacco companies, he argued, were falsely advertising their products. Instead of the potentially fatal health hazards and addictive menaces that they were, cigarettes were presented, in effect, as healthful, life-improving, and alluring by the companies. Under the leadership of FTC Chairman Pertshuk, the Commission issued a proposed regulation requiring the companies to clearly label their products as serious threats to health. Although Congress responded angrily and vindictively toward the FTC, the House and Senate were nevertheless forced to deal with the issue. In consultation with their tobacco allies, congressional leaders negotiated softer language and enacted legislation that for the first time mandated that the industry warn users of their products.

The most dramatic and successful example of venue-shifting occurred when the courts in the United States became deeply involved in the controversy. Cigarette manufacturers were sued a number of times beginning in the 1940s by smokers (or their surviving family members) who developed terminal cancers as a result of smoking. But until the early 1990s the courts, in virtually every case, decided in favor of the industry. At first, the courts were unconvinced that the scientific evidence of cause (smoking) and effect (death) was sufficiently tight to warrant a decision in favor of the claimants. Ironically, the mandatory warning put on cigarette packages and advertising was subsequently used by the tobacco companies to convince the courts that smokers knew the harms of smoking and did not deserve payment from tobacco companies for their suffering. The string of losses by plaintiffs changed in the 1990s. Not only did a few plaintiffs succeed in court but a new set of actors brought a new and truly innovative approach to the courts that led the major tobacco companies in 1998 to agree to a series of actions intended to restrict smoking, especially by children.

While the episode is far too convoluted to explicate fully here, it illustrates the strategic importance coupling a new frame with a change in venue. The new frame in this case was provided by Mississippi Attorney-General Michael Moore who devised a novel ground on which to sue the tobacco corporations. Perhaps, he argued, smokers are to blame for their illnesses, given that they were warned of the health hazard caused by smoking. However, the state governments, which had to pay the health bill for many stricken smokers who could not otherwise afford medical care, were innocent third parties. As a result, he argued, the tobacco companies should reimburse state governments for the billions of dollars they spend on medical care for patients with smoking-related illnesses. Attorney-General Moore convinced most of the other 51 state attorneys-general (including the District of Columbia) to participate in this claim. Several factors led the companies to come to the bargaining table, including the increasingly negative climate of opinion toward the tobacco companies, their fear that more court losses were in the offing, and the damning revelation that that these corporations may intentionally have been spiking cigarettes with additional nicotine to increase addiction (and hence smoking). By 1998, a final, out-of-court settlement that constituted the most sweeping regulation of the industry ever was reached between the major manufacturers and the states. Many of the terms of the settlement were incorporated in the first and only international treaty on tobacco control, ratified in 2005, the Framework Convention on Tobacco Control, negotiated within the structure of the WHO.

Lesson 5. At its heart public policy is driven by politics, not scientific research

Maneuvering and deal-making is a fundamental element of gaining leverage and of creating majorities necessary for policy change in democracies. On the whole, this method of operating could not be further from that of medical researchers and other scientists, a fact that makes working across the two cultures of scientific research and politics especially challenging. Bridging this chasm requires policy elites and scientists whose research is policy-relevant to understand that the urgency of scientific results—even when decisive and clearly communicated, as argued above—is always tempered not only by the strength of the status quo but also by the need to create majorities for change. Policy change typically requires enormous political skill.

In tobacco control policy this point became clear very quickly. Tobacco farmers, for example, relied on tobacco-related products for their livelihood, and for a half-century growing tobacco was subsidized by the federal government. At the same time, by the 1990s, public opinion toward smoking grew increasingly negative, and government policy, especially at the state and local levels, was to discourage, if not regulate, tobacco use. The inconsistency in policy—subsidizing tobacco farmers while levying federal and state excise taxes on cigarettes in part to discourage smoking, for example—might be anathema to a logician (or a scientist) but is perfectly understandable as an expression of democratic politics. Eventually, the discrepancy became sufficiently glaring to require a political solution: Congress agreed to buy the farmers out. If they would agree to use their acreage for purposes other than growing tobacco, the growers would receive a large federal payment. Ten billion dollars were appropriated for this purpose with the result that the formidable tobacco coalition was weakened. The number of tobacco farmers dwindled and were no longer available to support the pro-tobacco cause, and, importantly, members of Congress from tobacco-growing states who had sided with the tobacco companies no longer had as compelling a reason to do so in the future. These officials now could be reelected without being pro-tobacco.

Lesson 6. New issues threaten existing political understandings and arrangements

Organizations and leaders who have become successful within existing arrangements have a stake in maintaining them. As a result, a new issue that could jeopardize standing agreements, on which existing leaders and organizations rely, typically requires not only new leadership but new leadership of a particular kind, that of the policy entrepreneur. Such a person understands politics but is not wedded to the status quo and is exceedingly energetic, innovative, and driven. In a similar vein, even existing organizations that would seem to be "natural" allies to the new cause must be actively recruited, as their compass is calibrated to the status quo and not to the new issue and new frame.

In the case of tobacco control, the movement was blessed with a series of very successful policy entrepreneurs. None of them was as well known, well placed and capable as David A. Kessler. Kessler, a physician and attorney, was appointed by Republican President George W. H. Bush and reappointed by Democrat Bill Clinton to head the Food and Drug Administration. This bipartisan endorsement put him in a leadership position in the politics of tobacco control for many years. Kessler was no ordinary FDA administrator. He is an example of a quintessential policy entrepreneur. Talented, highly credentialed—with Ivy League law and medical degrees, as well as experience in government—he knew how creatively to use the powers of his position to bring about change. Kessler's accomplishment came to fruition over a number of years. Many of his ideas were incorporated in the 1998 tobacco agreement, discussed above. Over a decade after he left office, in 2009 Congress enacted legislation finally giving the Food and Drug Administration regulatory authority over nicotine, a policy change Kessler had championed for decades.

Just as new issues require new leaders who are not attached to the status quo, new issues are not necessarily embraced by existing organizations whose goals would seem to be consistent with the new issue. For almost every policy issue in the United States, groups are already organized that would seem to be, and often are, automatically interested in a matter that corresponds to their reason for existence. However, such groups must be convinced that the issue, like tobacco control by government, will work to serve their organization's interests. Moreover, such groups already have committed their resources and energies to certain reform programs and are less available for new approaches. Old line health organizations like the American Cancer Society, American Heart Association (AHA) or American Lung Association (ALA), which have missions which are not coterminous with governmental regulation of smoking, were not initially at the forefront of this cause, though the ALA, for example, had sponsored ground-breaking research on the connection between smoking and lung cancer as early as the 1950s, and all of these groups saw smoking as a health hazard.

The important point here is that new organizations necessarily compete with existing organizations—even their seemingly "natural" allies—for attention, money, and time from the media, the public and policy elites. Moreover, innovative frames may occlude established ones that benefit existing organizations. As a result, those groups that may seem to be automatic allies cannot be taken for granted and must be convinced that their causes and organizations would be advanced by aligning with another. Apparently concerned that current donors may be offended by a campaign that directly attacked tobacco use and tobacco companies, the long-established societies were at first reluctant to take on the issue of governmental regulation. The American Medical Association, the leading association for practicing physicians in the United States, actually benefited from the patronage of tobacco companies in the 1950s and did not provide leadership on the harms of smoking.

Conclusion

Medical professionals and scientists need not become politicians to have significant influence in the policy process, but they need the tools and the flexibility to operate in a political, as opposed to a scientific, culture. In addition to understanding what those tools are and how they might be used, it is important to be aware that political power and effectiveness in policy processes for professionals stems largely from their standing in the eyes of the public. Public trust and respect is the root support for professionals in policymaking. Professional ethics and reputation are important. That trust is eroded when research scientists bend their results to please corporate sponsors or are paid large sums by the producers of pharmaceutical products they study. Such practices can weaken the stature of the profession and weaken scientists' role in public policy debates.[5]

Applying the political lessons above too literally could similarly harm the stature of scientists and medical professionals who are drafted into the political arena. In his discussion of issue framing, Brion J. Fox of the University of Wisconsin Comprehensive Cancer Center suggests that health policy professionals make certain to frame the issues they support in the context of their own values:

> [By framing] public health efforts in accordance with core ethical principles, the public health community can create more positive messages. ...Through the increased use of ethics in tobacco control, the public health community may be better positioned to claim the high road as the protector of the public's interests.
>
> ... people and movements are defined not solely by substance, but by how much the speaker's values resonate with the public. A truth spoken by a messenger who is not trusted will be disbelieved. If the tobacco control community is disbelieved, it may not be the result of being wrong, but rather from a failure to frame ourselves in such a way that our goals and our approaches resonate with the public.... [T]he tobacco control community should more proactively frame its actions and base that frame upon ethical principles (Fox 2005).

Medical and science professionals in good standing can take leadership roles in public policy, and they will increasingly be called upon to do so. As more medical and science initiatives find their way on to the public policy agenda, their expertise will be needed. Policy success, as the lessons above make clear, requires more than substantive, scientific knowledge. If science and medicine are to be incorporated properly and fully into public policy decisions, it is necessary not only for the public and their representatives to understand science. Scientists, too, will need to be politically literate and, at the same time, to perform in a way that strengthens the public's trust in them and in the integrity of their research.

---

[5] See *Good Work: When Excellence and Ethics Meet* (Gardner, Csikszentmihalyi, and Damon, 2001) for instructive case studies on the decline of ethics in some professions and the negative consequences that ensue.

References

Bachrach, Peter, and Morton S. Baratz. 1962. "Two Faces of Power." *The American Political Science Review* 56 (4):947-952.

Centers for Disease Control and Prevention. "History of the Surgeon General's Reports on Smoking and Health." http://www.cdc.gov/tobacco/data_statistics/sgr/history/index.htm(accessed August 7, 2009).

Centers for Disease Control and Prevention. 2006. *Morbidity and Mortality Weekly Report (MMWR).* 57(45):1226-1228.

Centers for Disease Control and Prevention. 2004. *The Health Consequences of Smoking: A Report of the Surgeon General.* Washington, DC: U.S. Department of Health and Human Services. http://www.cdc.gov/tobacco/data_statistics/sgr/2004/index.htm (accessed August 7, 2009).

Department of Health, Education, and Welfare. 1964. *Smoking and Health: Report of the Advisory Committee to the Surgeon General of the Public Health Service, Public Health Service.* Washington, DC: U.S. Department of Health, Education, and Welfare.

Engelhard, Carolyn L., Arthur Garson Jr, and Stan Dorn. 2009. "Reducing Obesity: Policy Strategies from the Tobacco Wars." http://www.urban.org/publications/411926.html (accessed August 9, 2009).

Fox, Brion J. 2005. "Framing Tobacco Control Efforts within an Ethical Context." *Tobacco Control* 14 (Supplement 2):ii38-ii44.

Fritschler, A. Lee, and Catherine E. Rudder. 2007. *Smoking and Politics.* Prentice Hall.

Frontline, PBS. 1998. "Interview with Gerald Huber." *Inside the Tobacco Deal.* http://www.pbs.org/wgbh/pages/frontline/shows/settlement/interviews/huber.html.

Gardner, Howard, Mihaly Csikszentmihalyi, and William Damon. 2001. *Good Work : When Excellence and Ethics Meet.* New York: Basic Books.

Kingdon, John W. 2002. *Agendas, Alternatives, and Public Policies*, 2nd Edition. Longman.

Majone, Giandomenico. 1992. *Evidence, Argument, and Persuasion in the Policy Process.* Yale University Press.

National Research Council. 1986. *Environmental Tobacco Smoke: Measuring Exposures and Assessing Health Effects.* Washington DC: National Academy Press.

Olson, Mancur. 1965. *The Logic of Collective Action: Public Goods and the Theory of Groups.* Cambridge, MA: Harvard University Press.

Rudder, Catherine E. 2008. "Private Governance as Public Policy: A Paradigmatic Shift." *The Journal of Politics* 70 (4):899-913.

Schattschneider, E. E. 1960. *Semisovereign People.* Holt, Rinehart and Winston.

III. Decentralization and Health Care Delivery

Regionalization of the Public Health System and New Governance Models for Healthcare: The Stroke Network Case in Italy

Domenica Farinella, *University of Cagliari*
Pietro Saitta, *University of Messina*
Guido M. Signorino, *University of Messina*

Introduction

Recent Developments of the Italian National Health System

Italy has had a predominantly public national health system since the 1970s. Health has an important symbolic value for the public; therefore, healthcare is a fundamental element in political consensus and public spending (Sharpe 1988; Pavolini 2009). In 1992, Italy went through a series of legal scandals (the famous *Mani pulite* inquiry), remedied through drastic public administration system reform.[1] This gave local government unprecedented autonomy in public service management, including healthcare. The process of devolution took place during a time of limited government revenue and local expenditure (France 2008). As a consequence, the main objectives over the last decade have been to control spending, introduce managed competition in private and public sectors, and ration health services (Vicarelli and Pavolini 2009).

Currently, national and regional political decisions are made during specific negotiation sessions (*Conferenze Permanenti* or Permanent Conferences) rather than in the parliament or by the ministries (France and Taroni 2005). In this framework, the ministers are neutral, acting to uphold constitutional laws and enact flexible guidelines to be locally implemented (Vicarelli 2005). As a result, there is a considerable lack of consistency in regional budget performance and medical care quality (Kazepov and Genova 2005; Cartocci 2007).

The administrative decentralization and the New Public Management inspired new public reform processes (Hood 1991; Box 1999; Stivers 2003). The Italian administrative system, compared to the French formalistic and *etatist* tradition, was characterized by a bureaucratic-functional model (Cerase 1990; Battistelli 1998), which assigns a primary role to the State (Cassese 1977; Fedele 1998). During the post-war years, this model, combined with the State's growing intervention in the economy, caused administrative expansion into the most productive areas of the country. In the southern regions, public interventionism followed a model of "development without autonomy" (Trigilia 1992; Putnam 1993), characterized by unemployment, lower wages, and a weaker entrepreneurial system. The public sector expanded, replacing private enterprises, and became central to the regional employment practices. This expansion allowed for political patronage in recruitment processes. The public sector in southern Italy became the milieu where electoral support was exchanged for jobs (Cerase 1990) and corporate

---

[1] The administrative hierarchical order in Italy consists of state, region, province, and local council (comune).

interests were upheld (Farinella 2005). This harmed the public administration effectiveness in the south, due to the inability to provide quality services, and created an administrative dualism between the north and the south.

The national health system, one of the most important public sectors, was not immune to these practices. To switch from the bureaucratic model to the managerial and privatized one, the process of "corporatization" of health structures was initiated. Older Local Health Units (USL or *Unità Sanitarie Locali*), hierarchically included in the broader regional administrative system, were transformed into Local Health Companies (ASL or *Aziende Sanitarie Locali*) and larger hospitals were broken down into Hospital Companies (AO or *Aziende Ospedaliere*). ASL and AO exist as separate legal organizations and have more autonomy compared to the rest of the administrative system (Anessi-Pessina and Cantù 2004; Balduzzi and Di Gaspare 2001).

The governance of the Italian health system can be described as follows:

• *Higher level*: Health Ministry, Parliament, and Government (responsible for programming and establishing the national health agenda (PSN—*Piano Sanitario Nazionale* or National Sanitary Plan)

• *Middle level*: The regions (responsible for actuating the PSN, with independent legislative powers, spending powers, and the power to appoint health management and staff)

• *Lower level*: Local Health Services (responsible for maintaining relations with general practitioners, corporatized hospitals who sell their services, and other public and private health structures inside and outside the region).

The public make their financial contribution to the national health system by paying national and local taxes or by contributing a fee. This "ticket" varies regionally (Ferrera 2006). The term "regionalization" sums up the Italian regions' effort toward legislative independence and services reorganization.

This research was developed within the context of this differentiation process with the aim of understanding the reasons for differences in the development of basic healthcare services, such as cerebrovascular stroke networks in Italy.

The Stroke Network in the Italian Regions: Design and Implementation Problems

Longitudinal population studies and the "Permanent Conference for the Relationships Between the State, the Regions, and the Independent Provinces of Trento and Bolzano (2005)" recognize that "the cerebrovascular stroke represents one of the most important health issues, and is the primary cause of permanent disability, the second most important etiology of dementia, and (in Italy) the third major reason for mortality resulting in significant socio-economic impacts" (Ricci et al. 1991; D'Alessandro et al. 1992; Lauria et al. 1995; Di Carlo et al. 2003). The conference evaluated the evidence that early intervention and rehabilitation improves all outcomes in stroke victims (Langhorne and Dennis 2004; Drummond et al. 2005; Candelise et al. 2007; Saka et al. 2009). On February 3, 2005, a State–Regional agreement promoted the creation of stroke treatment networks and gave hospitals the authority to establish stroke units (SUs) using dedicated and multidisciplinary treatment teams.

The stroke network is built around the patient. General practitioners are responsible for providing the patient at risk of stroke (due to smoking and obesity) with educational materials and lifestyle modifications (such as regular physical activity). In the event of an emergency, a simple telephone notification activates the stroke network and ensures prompt patient access to treatment using standardized protocols (the Cincinnati Stroke Scale and the Glasgow Coma Scale). Rapid recovery in an SU during the acute phase allows patients to be monitored in a hospital bed, to have integrated treatment, and an early opportunity to start the rehabilitation. It also helps to increase the number of patients eligible for thrombolysis. After discharge from the hospital, patients are enrolled in a rehabilitation facility designed to reintegrate them into society. A schematic representation of the whole process is shown in Figure 1.

Nevertheless, the transition from *best evidence* to *best practice*, with the structural change development necessary for patient care, is problematic and requires a shared approach at different organizational and patient care levels (Grol and Grimshaw 2003).

Figure 1. The Stroke Network: An Integrated Process

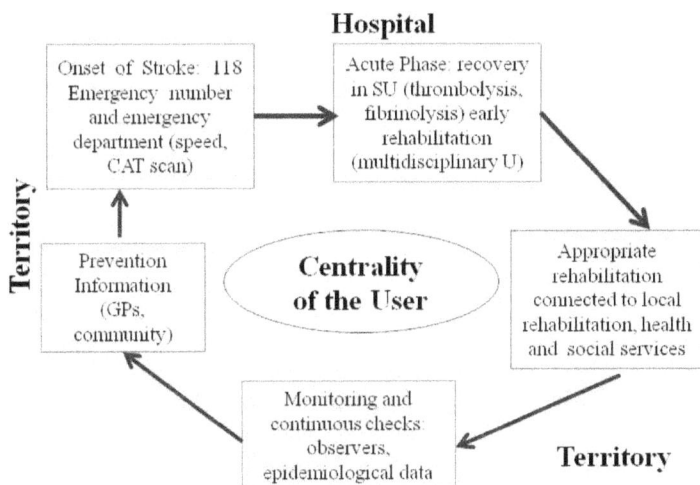

Source: Authors' elaboration based on the State–Regional Agreement (2005).

The Research Project on Hospital Admission for Stroke Patients in Italy (PROSIT) compared outcomes and performance quality between SUs and non-specialized general medical units (GW). This study included facilities that treated more than 50 stroke patients per year (Bersano et al. 2006). Sixty-eight SUs and 677 GW were selected, of which the SU showed a significantly better performance. SU prevalence in Italy accounted for 8% of admission, in contrast to countries like Great Britain where SUs are operative in 83% of hospitals (Rudd et al. 2005). Also, SUs are more prevalent in the Center-North of Italy (Figure 2).

Figure 2. Distribution of Stroke Units in Italy

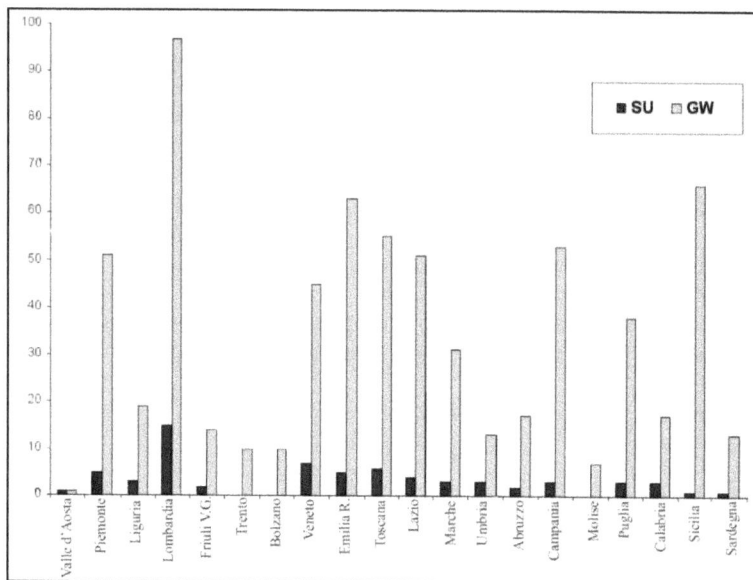

Source: Bersano et al. (2006).

Recent research on 14 regions, by Ferro et al. (2008), has confirmed this uneven distribution, including full operability only available in a few regions.

Methods

Our study was supported by the Center for Health Management and Prevention of Diseases (*Centro Controllo e Prevenzione delle Malattie* or CCM) and the Health Ministry. The study compares six regions' organizational models to develop guidance for regions which are suffering from slower implementation of the stroke treatment networks. Different models were considered (Glaser and Strauss 1967) for the study. Qualitative tools, particularly semi-structured in-depth interviews and focus groups, were used (King, Keohan, and Verba 1994; Krueger 1994; Liamputtong and Ezzy 2005). The selected models compensated for the inappropriateness of quantitative tools in measuring the dynamics of an ongoing process such as a stroke network (Granovetter 1973; 2000; Schein 1985; North 1990; Alvesson and Berg 1992; Lanzalaco 1995; Hatch 1997). To achieve an in-depth analysis, we concentrated on a limited number of regions and stakeholders who play strategic roles.

The selected six regions comprised the following:

- Campania and Calabria have minimal implementation of the network, with one stroke network still at the planning stage and only a few SUs.
- Marche and Toscana have a moderate implementation level of the network planned, but this is not currently a functioning network. SUs are unevenly distributed in the regions.
- Lombardy and Piedmont have a high implementation level.

For each region, core "representative" interviewers were selected. The "representative" included a lead neurologist who was knowledgeable of the health organization's internal dynamics in the region.

Data on each region's stroke network structure and relevant legislations were compiled first. Between 6 and 12 people from each region were interviewed for a total of 52 in-depth interviews (Table 1). The original intent was to include a politician specializing in health (a local government health councilor or his delegate), a regional technical director, head of health planning, a technical director for regional health agencies (where present), up to two hospitals' administrators (ASL, hospital, polyclinic), a hospital health director, a director of an SU or (if not available) a neurology department chair, a dean of the medical faculty, and a president of the Medical Association (the latter two were considered as part of vested interest stakeholders). Some potential interviewees declined to participate (Table 1). A larger number of stakeholders in Lombardy and Campania volunteered to participate and were included in the interviews.

Table 1. Distribution of the Participants by Region

Region	No. of Interviewees	Not Participating
Calabria	6	Dean of Faculty; Councilor; SU Director
Campania	12	Councilor
Lombardy	8	Councilor
Tuscany	9	Dean of Faculty
Marche	8	Councilor
Piedmont	9	Regional Technical Director
Total	52	

A "flexible" approach toward the interviews was adopted. These interviews preceded the creation of six focus groups (one for each region). The focus group participants were located using social networks. Interviewees were asked to indicate one or more individuals of particular relevance within the regional systems who could be contacted to participate in the focus group discussions (Table 2).

Table 2. Composition of the Focus Groups per Region

Role within the Health System	Calabria	Campania	Marche	Tuscany	Lombardy	Piedmont
Head of Regional Planning	1		1	2	1	1
Head of Regional Health Agency		1	1	1		1
Head of Stroke Network	1	1	1	1	1	1
Head of Emergencies	1	1	1	2	1	1
Head of Rehabilitation Network	1	1	2	1	2	1
Head of Patients' Association (ALICE)	1	1	1	1	1	1
Head of Cardiology Network	1	1		1	1	1
Head of Oncology Network		2	1	1		1
Health or General Director of ASL or Hospital	1			3	1	1
General Practitioner	1		2	2	2	2
Total	8	8	10	15	10	11

A total of 114 individuals were interviewed between the focus groups and interviewees, all of whom were responsible for:

• principal care networks (oncology, cardiology, emergency, stroke, rehabilitation),

• different local health organizations (general directors of ASLs or hospitals),

• regional planning (regional directors or regional health organization directors responsible for planning and/or the organization of health resources),

• representing general practitioner associations.

All information obtained from the two interviews was analyzed using Atlas.ti software as described in the grounded theory research methodology (Glaser and Strauss 1967).

Results

The study showed that, regardless of the number of functioning SUs in the area, all regions are having difficulty in activating stroke networks. The reasons common to all regions were (1) budget constraints (especially in the southern territories) due to national and regional financial restrictions, (2) lack of communication between the health sectors and the inner cities and suburbs, (3) competition between doctors and disciplines, (4) competition between hospitals, and (5) lack of patient and public interest on the issue under study.

The northern regions of Italy are in a more advanced stage of implementation than the southern regions. However, many problems which are common to the Italian healthcare system are much more complex than the stereotyped North–Centre–South divide. Results summarizing different institutional variables and the status of the local stroke network implementation phases are displayed in Table 3. Additional information is presented in the Appendix at the end of this paper.

Table 3. Principal Characteristics of Regional Health Systems

Region	Model	Characteristics	Stroke Network
Lombardy	Competitive	- Low centrality in the region. - Widespread presence of private operators. - Independent organization and design of facilities. - Policy collaboration. -Competition between hospitals/clinics, independently of their public or private status.	The distributed network is in place.
Campania	Formalistic-bureaucratic	- Separation between region and territory. - Formal centralism of the region, excessive legislation. - Dualism between coastal and in-land areas. - Formalized system of control and monitoring, absence of shared protocols between region and local actors.	The network exists on a formal level, bureaucratic difficulties hampering implementation. Greater success in suburban areas.
Calabria	Individualistic-fragmentary	- Individualism. - Fragmentation, politicization. - Lack of cooperation. - Economic emergence.	Delays in decision making (regulations approved in mid-2009). Early stages of network formation, centered mostly on the creation of an SU.
Marche	Spontaneous-fragmentary (reactive)	-Insufficient coordination, in spite of regional management and monitoring. -Spontaneism. -Moderate resistance to changing of doctors.	Absence of a stroke network. Little coordination between acute and post-acute.
Tuscany	Redistributive-egalitarian	- Centrality and dirigisme of the region (incorporation of the territory into planning). - Institutionalized collaboration of policies. - "Horizontal" approach to skills (diffusion of practical knowledge on all levels). - Tendency toward public sector (subordinate of private).	Stroke network organized from grassroots and on individual initiatives. In a formative phase due to unresolved decisions on the models to follow.
Piedmont	Redistributive-egalitarian	- Centrality of the region and the public sector. - Important participation of volunteers and associations (often "steered" and run by physicians).	Stroke network in the process of being consolidated, but good attention to all network phases.

Even the more advanced regions, such as Lombardy, Tuscany, and Piedmont, are having difficulty managing the entire implementation of the network. The primary obstacle stems from the lack of communication between health and social services in the post-acute phase of the stroke and the lack of adequate interface processes and guidelines.

Discussion

While the Italian health system is becoming increasingly regionalized (Maino 1999; Maino 2001; Taroni 2007), it is possible to pinpoint common trends. First, there is a transition toward networks serving major chronic diseases (oncology network, cardiology, etc.) and the integration of services tailored to community health (Ranci 2006). The stroke example demonstrates the tendency of developing grassroot networks based on cooperation and collaboration among experts who work in the regions and territories (usually through commissions and study groups).

The developing health service network model implies that the national health system is being transitioned in favor of a more local and integrated model (Cepiku 2006; Martelli 2007). Stakeholder support and accountability become important elements to ensure accreditation and quality control.

A managed healthcare system, which started in the 80s, has resulted in greater budgeting and resource allocation in an attempt to improve effectiveness and efficiency. Downsizing and rationing in hospital care stems from the need to reduce costs and demonstrates the necessity to transition traditional healthcare concepts to meet local and more individualized services. Regulatory decentralization, social-health integration, territory centralization, administrative competition, healthcare corporatization, public hospital liberalization, increased fiscal responsibility, and network organization are common to all Italian regions (Vicarelli 2005; Ferrera 2006). An analysis of the differences in the stroke Framework Agreement implementation has underlined the centrality of path dependence and institutional factors (North 1990), along with the organizational design of the stroke network. This study has attempted to highlight how some of these characteristics result in different outcomes for stroke network organization. For example, the centrality of the organizational principle of equity in Tuscany and of competition in Lombardy reflects a diametrically opposite approach to networks. In the Tuscany case, it is hierarchical; the network nodes are "incorporated" into public policy objectives but have little autonomy. Alternatively, in the Lombardy case, the network is defined by the course it takes when different network nodes are competing with each other.

Therefore, institutional and cultural characteristics can work both as delaying and enhancing factors for each implementation strategy. For example, the formal and individualistic culture of Calabrian medical specialists and regional stakeholders creates limits and fragmentation, thus hindering cooperation which is so vital to the smooth running of the network. Conversely, the association and volunteer culture present in Marche, Piedmont, and Tuscany represents a particularly useful resource that, nevertheless, is often not adequately appreciated and can also become a constraint (i.e., the volunteer ambulance service in Tuscany).

As has been highlighted in Table 2, the formation of local stroke networks reflects the organizational characteristics of each region and is the result of institutional isomorphic change (Fennell 1980; DiMaggio and Powell 1983). In the least developed regions, where the tendency to reproduce models applied somewhere else is greater, unintended consequences can result. Lombardy has created a model based on public and private competition. Piedmont has generated another model founded on principles of cooperation and public needs. These are very different models that might not be transferrable to other regions with different socio-economic structures.

Stroke networks are less likely to advance when stakeholders are unable to combine general principles and "reality." Under these circumstances, differences and strains are liable to arise and should be considered with a debate over how to best deliver quality care.

Conclusions and Policy Implications

Generally, the best working model is one that closely reflects the healthcare system needs within which it is developed. When there is a lack of coordination between institutional actors and professionals, stroke networks are unlikely to be supported and built. For this reason, policies should be framed within the culture, values, and norms of the local social and health context. Our study shows that, even in the most developed regions, interfaces between different networks are critical. We have identified the most common causes of disconnect that should be carefully evaluated and addressed in the process of planning healthcare networks:

1. The type of conflict arising from the relationship between health services and the regional administration is a result of services and managing costs (Merton 1949; Crozier 1964; Simon 1955; Elston 1992; Hood 1995; Gauld 2001). The southern regions such as Calabria and Campania, with a bureaucratic model of health organization and lower levels of administrative performance, are those where the delay is more evident. Administrative "red tape" (Bozeman 2000) generates fragmentation, redundancy, individualism, and lack of communication. Remediation consists of improved communications and care providers' participation in the decision processes (Weick 1969).

2. The relationship between hospitals and territories involves hospital physicians and general practitioners (Maarse, Mur-Veeman, and Tijssen 1990; Marshall 1998; Le Doare, Banerjee, and Oldfield 2009). As shown by the Lombardy, Piedmont, and, partially, Tuscany cases, the most advanced stroke networks are those developed after the reorganization of a "territorial network" of general practitioners (through the use of electronic patient files and databases). Physician participation helps the network to stay focused on the territorial networks rather than only on the acute phases of stroke treatment.

3. The conflict/competition between non-university and university hospitals stems from their different roles in the healthcare system (care-giving versus research/training) and the differences in their respective status (Choi, Allison, and Munson 1985; Campbell, Weissman, and Blumenthal 1997; Sohn 1997; Editorial 2001). The most successful stroke networks are those operating in areas where these conflicts are less pronounced and include two main strategies: non-university hospitals providing training and internships (as in Lombardy).

4. The specialization and multidisciplinary approach to medical practice can lead different medical specialties and different organizational systems to compete with each other (Freidson 1970; Abbott 1988; Nancarrow and Borthwick 2005). The Tuscany case reveals the negative effects of the lack of balance between specialization and multidisciplinary practice in organizations. Neurologists and political actors do not develop a common vision of the role of integrated care within the health organization and do not rely on each other. Thus, integrated stroke assistance fails, despite the otherwise good performance in the region.

Competitive relationships can be overcome by improving communication and education processes. The analysis of successful cases (e.g., the hospitals of Melegnano in Lombardy, Benevento in Campania, and San Benedetto in the Marche) shows that improvements are noted when

- management is devoted to a cooperative style of leadership, involving professionals who take their responsibilities seriously;
- "departmental" and multidisciplinary hospital organizations embrace collaboration and exchanges, also valuing and acknowledging the role of nurses and paramedics.

In Italy, there is a lack of acknowledgement that stroke is a "time-dependent" disease. Neurologists should lead innovation in this field, in a cooperative framework with other specialties.

The analysis shows that stroke networks that work within the existing infrastructure are the most effective. For example, in Lombardy construction of the stroke network took place after the emergency network had been created; the stroke network is also "emergency-oriented." Alternatively, in Tuscany and Piedmont territorial services were developed, and the stroke network is mostly oriented toward rehabilitation and the integration between hospital and social services. Goals should be set in each region for improving communication problems and collaborative practices (D'Albergo 2002).

To conclude, the focus of this contribution is on Italy. However, the experience of this country provides an insight into the internal dynamics of publicly funded health organizations facing scarce resources. This analysis, within the path dependency framework, demonstrated how the shift from account management to "territorial health governance" takes place in different areas. Our analysis shows the importance of overcoming a rigid burcaucratic management in favor of shared and localized practices. Finally, reflecting on the Italian case can be interesting to understand not only the problems related to this topic, but also the general problems of healthcare systems in Europe.

Appendix A: Regional Reports

Appendix A summarizes regional interviews and focus groups discussions. The interested reader can better understand local contexts and the polymorphism of the Italian Health System, where differentiation is much more complex than the North–South divide.

1. Calabria

The Calabrian Health Service is in a nascent state of development. The region is temporarily administered by a commissioner, and an austere financial recovery plan is expected. In this region's health service, there are a large number of small hospitals that will be closed due to rationing of resources and reorganization of hospital services. According to the interviewed regional directors, the closure of these minor hospitals is being met with strong political and social objections. For medical workers, the widespread welfare culture present in today's society overburdens hospitals with unnecessary work, weighing them down with the treatment of less serious cases that could be directed to local facilities. Overall, the interviewees reinforced that, due to the financial deficit, the margins to move within health policies are greatly reduced and simply focused on expenditure restraint with the reduction of social services. The scarce attention to patients' needs and lack of epidemiological data during the planning stage could, over time, slow down the overall system reorganization. These problems are common to Calabria and Campania. The interviewed doctors stated that within health facilities, there is a prevailing attitude of isolation and lack of communication, promoting fragmentation and poor cooperation. In a similar way, the regional and hospital managers observed that a closed, individualistic attitude and lack of teamwork spirit is characteristic of the specialists who consider such activities as a threat to their own power.

In 2009, a committee decision was made to develop an integrated healthcare program. The network is still to be fully realized (prevention, hospitalization, and post-hospital treatment). At the moment, the greatest efforts are being concentrated on the care of acute patients with the creation of SUs in some of the largest hospitals. Most of these initiatives come from the grassroots and are the work of health directors at the request of neurologists. The new units are created by adapting existing hospital space and by reassigning the staff trained by neurologists who are in charge of the facility.

2. Campania

The health system in Campania presents elements of territorial dualism. On the one hand, there are Benevento and Avellino, smaller mountain provinces, with low population size, low crime rates, and discreet health service management including some areas of excellence. On the other hand, the coastal areas (Naples, Caserta, and part of Salerno) have urban congestion, high population density, and an inefficient distribution of health facilities. In Naples, there are some old and obsolete hospitals that have a long history and are therefore difficult to close (like the one in the "Spanish Quarters"). There is a permanent state of emergency and management difficulties, along with fragmentation, individualism, private healthcare, and social conflicts. From the interviews, it emerges that social conflict is reflected on different levels:

- Between the users, reasoning in selfish and free-riding ways, with an attitude geared toward consumption of services and not the collective good (Donolo 2001).
- Between the users and health organizations. Free-riding users with a high degree of mistrust toward the institution trap the hospitals in a situation of emergency. This has become routine, making planning, project creation, and improving the quality of services very difficult.
- Between health facilities and regional administrations who do not communicate. This creates a divide between what is defined by law and what is actually accomplished. Local operators complain about formal management decisions from above regarding the means, resources, and procedures with which they should accomplish their objectives. As a consequence, and in the absence of inspections, there is a tendency not to execute many directives.

As Vicarelli and Pavolini (2009) observed, Campania is distinguished by excessive legislation from adjacent regions. The effect is a phenomenon of de-empowerment when the administration's authority is exhausted during the decision-making process (Merton 1949).

Moreover, this tendency shows how similar Campania is to other regions. Campania has proven incapable of managing losses from the economic deficit, despite the ample number of plans and measures for repayments (France 2008; Vicarelli and Pavolini 2009). The stroke network issue is symbolic of this. Currently, there is only one regional act, which resulted from the work of a panel of experts convened in 2005, defining the network and approach to care by promoting SU adoption. None of the recommendations were enacted, with Naples unable to carry out thrombolysis, and no truly functional SUs.

The Rummo Hospital in Benevento illustrates an interesting experience. Thanks to the presence of neurologists from outside the region, a stroke unit has been created and a makeshift network is being sketched out. This mitigates the regional shortcomings and lack of financial resources through cooperation between the 118 emergency line manager and several rehabilitation facilities. With just a few modifications, they have equipped several rooms, bought medical equipment and monitored beds, trained operators and staff, and created a patient triage in collaboration with a large, local, and private rehabilitation facility. In Benevento, the neurologists are responsible for finding a place in a suitable rehabilitation center for their patients, even though this increases their workload. In this way they compensate for the inadequate links between the hospital and rehabilitation facilities.

According to the doctors and even some regional managers, epidemiological data have no effect on health planning. Despite the strong regional incidence of stroke, the latest health plans show that there has been a decreased attention for this disease. Some hospital managers and doctors complain that there are major bureaucratic hurdles for establishing an SU.

3. Marche

The Marche region has a high degree of consensus for health planning. This has been achieved through the region's inclusive and collaborative project planning methods. Planning for stroke treatment was first considered in the 2003–2006 Health Plan, and today there are six functioning SUs in the area. The board, responsible for collecting scientific evidence and studying best practices, was made up of a group of regional stroke experts, consultants from the relevant disciplines (accident and emergency, internal medicine, neurology, and neuroradiology), and nurses. Regional approval for the SUs will take at least three years.

However, since 2003 the S. Benedetto hospital has been organizing its own SU in accordance with the regional planning. At S. Benedetto, the innovation was the direct result of collaboration between the local manager of the neurology division and the general hospital administrators. It was recommended to send the SU planner to Niguarda in Milan (one of the most advanced hospitals in the country) to study their organizational approach. Small donations for buying old but efficient equipment have allowed a neurologist group to become familiar with treatment techniques, conduct research, and publish findings. The experience in S. Benedetto reinforces how motivation and relationships can transcend organizational obstacles. Although the Marche region has limited resources, it seems to have fewer conflicts and a tendency toward cooperation.

4. Tuscany

The Tuscan healthcare system provides a good quality of medical care. Regional health plans are primarily directed toward the therapeutic treatment of strokes, but implementation levels within the network are average. The rationing of healthcare has been underway for some time, thus closing smaller hospitals. This has been made possible through a model of governance centralizing regional control and planning practices. Specifically, Tuscany has put into practice a model of institutionalized planning, and the principal stakeholders were included into the planning system.

Stakeholder interests are channeled and enhanced into a common cognitive framework, geared toward equity and universal performance. Institutions such as the Health Society (a permanent connection between regions and mayors), the Regional Health Council (providing institutional representation to specialists), or the mechanism of wide areas (normalizing the relationships between hospitals) are able to define the formal planning process and directions. The stakeholder interests are represented and can lead to the collective good. This produces less conflict, making it possible to reorganize hospitals by relocating facilities and allowing quality treatment throughout Tuscany.

Formally, there are 14 hospitals that treat about a quarter of the 10,000 annual stroke cases in the area. However, as outlined by the interviewees, this network is not structured. A network requires stable organizational and functional ties between the territorial services, emergency services, and hospitals. As with other regions, problems with local rehabilitation services still exist.

Practitioners and representatives from scientific associations together with institutional actors are "social partners," directing the planning and care process. Social partners are primarily made up of patient groups and their families. This model does not envision the availability of multidisciplinary facilities, employing dedicated professionals, but rather includes different members of the professional team (each from their own departments) able to intervene simultaneously. Thus SUs will be necessary in some but not all instances.

A general regional feature is the implementation of experimental post-stroke rehabilitation such as "adapted physical activity," consisting of individual rehabilitation projects that last for one or two years. These projects use approved public exercise facilities and try to guarantee rehabilitation continuity.

Although the subject creates much interest, the region faces certain limits. First, the emergency system, and the stroke call 118 line in particular, has too many volunteers and a high turnover rate. This makes it difficult to train staff and help them acquire necessary skills. These limitations affect the quality and outcomes of the interventions. Some neurologists have noted that, because strokes are silent, they can remain undiagnosed. Patients are often ignored in favor of those with less serious and more obvious problems. Training of personnel represents a major limitation in the Tuscan healthcare system.

5. Lombardy

Lombardy maintains a regional healthcare system that combines *network organization* and *competition*. They have a systemic approach for treatment of different diseases. For example, strokes are not treated by sector, but fall within a wide network of treatment for cerebro-cardiovascular diseases. This allows for resources to be used in the most efficient way.

The region leaves much of the organization of services up to the local hospitals, thus stimulating a sense of competition for the creation of new initiatives. This allows for experimentation with good practices within certain local areas. Each hospital is given full autonomy over implementation. This encourages competition in the search for best practices. Hospitals are motivated to present studies of effective and good treatment outcomes while competing for regional research funding.

For strokes, the hospital in Lecco is testing out a model to rationalize the emergency system and monitor response times in four peripheral provinces. Together, the Melegnano Hospital, Humanitas, and other facilities have obtained funding for a project for primary and secondary stroke prevention involving providers and families. This cooperation to identify good practices helps hospitals to develop autonomy, project planning, and managerial/relational skills. Further, since these practices require negotiation and sharing, they have a better chance of success and of producing organizational learning processes (Bifulco 1996). The competition between facilities to implement research projects is a strong innovation mechanism (Donolo and Fichera 1988). Small projects funding is very competitive because of scarce resources and penalizes the more peripheral hospitals. Compared to excellent public and private facilities, these hospitals cannot guarantee quality of services because of limited resources, a major limitation for expanding stroke networks (Jommi and Del Vecchio 2004; Pezzini 2005).

The decision-making process is managed by a working group made up of experts and actors involved in healthcare. Teamwork and regular consultation encourage the creation of common frames of action (D'Albergo 2002). This has also been the case for stroke treatment. The commission for cerebro-cardiovascular disease composed of experts and professionals from public and private health sectors, using epidemiological data and clinical evidence, has developed a set of guidelines, unique in that neither the number of regional SUs nor their locations have been decided beforehand. The stroke network is defined by indicators using timing, protocols, and telemedicine where particular specialists are unavailable.

The emergency system in Lombardy demonstrates excellent implementation and is well developed to handle stroke.

6. Piedmont

Piedmont is advanced in the deliberative process but suffers a delay in implementing an integrated network. Since 2005, the region has been strongly committed to the implementation of the guidelines, even though inefficiencies remain, linked to the limited numbers of SUs and post-acute healthcare facilities. Nevertheless, according to the interviewees, the regional healthcare issue is characterized by the centrality of "local" activities set up by facilities scattered over a wide area and subject to the demands of small local communities. This situation is fairly common and has led to the consolidation of local practices and culture.

"The self-sufficiency of services," as one witness describes, appears to be a feature common to healthcare managers and professionals who have difficulty teaching staff to render stroke care services. The decisions, according to one witness, are driven by concerns for regulations (Ross 1967).

The diffusion of new knowledge and skills even on peripheral levels can make up for the lack of specialized facilities. There is a skeptical vision of SUs (Blower and Au 1979; Andrews et al. 1981; Stroke Unit Trialist's Collaboration 2001). Other obstacles are more objective and linked to tight budgets or lack of personnel. For example, the speed (about 18 months) with which a hospital such as Le Molinette set up its SU can only be fully understood in the light of the availability of resources.

In spite of all difficulties, Piedmont is characterized by the collaborative way in which decisions are made. The main decision facilitator seems to be the Regional Agency for Health Services (Aress), which coordinates the working groups' activities. The agency creates groups responsible for particular areas (diseases, issues linked to prevention, etc.). In the case of stroke, there are representatives from the health department, nurses, GPs, and physiatrists. This inclusive approach has fostered a greater sense of involvement and participation.

The decision-making processes are not limited to the work of the commission. Instead, as one of the political witnesses observed, regional health plans are the fruit of political debates in which the participation of patients' associations is fundamental.

References

Abbott, A.D. 1988. *The System of Professions: An Essay on the Division of Expert Labor.* Chicago: University of Chicago Press.

Accordo Tra il Ministro della Salute. 2005. "Le Regioni e le Province Autonome di Trento e Bolzano del 3 Febbraio 2005." *Linee di Indirizzo per la Definizione del Percorso Assistenziale ai Pazienti con Ictus Cerebrale.* http://www.governo.it/backoffice/allegati/24489-2386.pdf.

Alvesson, M., and P.O. Berg. 1992. *Corporate Culture and Organizational Symbolism.* Berlin: Walter de Gruyter & Co.

Andrews, K., J.C. Brocklehurst, B. Richards, et al. 1981. "The Rate and Recovery from Stroke and its Measurement." *International Rehabilitation Medicine* 3: 151-161.

Anessi-Pessina, E., and E. Cantù. 2004. *L'aziendalizzazione della Sanità in Italia. Rapporto OASI 2004.* Egea: Milano.

Balduzzi, R., and G. Di Gaspare. 2001. *L'aziendalizzazione nel D.Lgs. 229/99.* Milano: Giuffré.

Battistelli, F. 1998. *Burocrazia e Mutamento.* Milano: FrancoAngeli.

Bersano, A., L. Candelise, R. Sterzi, G. Micieli, M. Gattinoni, A. Morabito, and the PROSIT Study Group. 2006. "Stroke Unit Care in Italy. Results from PROSIT (Project on Stroke Services in Italy). A Nationwide Study." *Neurological Sciences* 27: 332-339.

Bifulco, L. 1996. *L'apprendimento Organizzativo nei Servizi Socio-Sanitari. Pratiche di Cambiamento, Problemi e Possibilità.* Milano: FrancoAngeli.

Blower, P., and S. Au. 1979. "A Stroke Unit in a General Hospital: The Greenwich Experience." *British Medical Journal* 2: 644-649.

Box, R.C. 1999. "Running Government Like a Business: Implications for Public Administration Theory and Practice." *American Review of Public Administration* 29 (1): 19-43.

Bozeman, B. 2000. *Bureaucracy and Red Tape.* Upper Saddle River: Prentice-Hall Publishing.

Campbell, E.G., J.S. Weissman, and D. Blumenthal. 1997. "Relationship between Market Competition and the Activities and Attitudes of Medical School Faculty." *Journal of the American Medical Association* 278 (3): 222-226.

Candelise, M., M. Gattinoni, A. Bersano, G. Micieli, R. Sterzi, and A. Morabito. 2007. "Stroke-unit Care for Acute Stroke Patients: An Observational Follow-Up Study." *The Lancet* 369: 254-255.

Cartocci, R. 2007. *Mappe del Tesoro. Atlante del Capitale Sociale in Italia.* Bologna: Il Mulino.

Cassese, S. 1977. *Questione Amministrativa e Questione Meridionale.* Milano: Giuffré.

Cepiku, D. 2006. "Definizioni e Modelli di Public Governance." In *Managerialità, Innovazione e Governance*, eds. M. Meneguzzo, D. Cepiku, and E. De Filippo. Roma: Aracne.

Cerase, F. 1990. *Un'amministrazione Bloccata.* Milano: FrancoAngeli.

Choi, T. Allison, and F. Munson. 1985. "Impact of Environment on State University Hospital Performance. An Explanatory Model." *Medical Care* 23 (7): 855-871.

Crozier, M. 1964. *The Bureaucratic Phenomenon.* London: Tavistock.

D'Albergo, E. 2002. "Modelli di Governance e Cambiamento Culturale: Le Politiche Pubbliche fra Mercato e Comunità." In *La cultura delle Amministrazioni, tra Retorica e Innovazione*, ed. F. Battistelli. Milano: FrancoAngeli, 71-90.

D'Alessandro, G., M. Di Giovanni, L. Roveyaz, et al. 1992. "Incidence and Prognosis of Stroke in the Valle D'Aosta, Italy, First-year Results of a Community-Based Study." *Stroke* 23: 1712-1715.

Di Carlo, A., M. Baldereschi, C. Gandolfo, et al. 2003 "Stroke in an Elderly Population: Incidence and Impact on Survival and Daily Function." *Cerebrovascular Diseases* 16: 141-150.

DiMaggio, P.J., and W.W. Powell. 1983. "The Iron Cage Revisited: Institutional Isomorphism and Collective Rationality in Organizational Fields." *American Sociological Review* 48: 147-160.

Donolo, C. 2001. *Disordine*. Roma: Donzelli.

Donolo, C., and F. Fichera. 1988. *Le vie dell'innovazione*. Milano: Feltrinelli.

Drummond, A.E.R., B. Pearson, N.B. Lincoln, and P. Berman. 2005. "Ten-year Follow-up of a Randomized Controlled Trial of a Stroke Rehabilitation Unit." *British Medical Journal* 331 (7515): 491-492.

Editorial. 2001. "Researcher, Clinician, or Teacher?" *Lancet* 357: 1543.

Elston, M.A. 1992. "The Politics of Professional Power: Medicine in a Changing Health Service." In *The Sociology of Health Service*, eds. J. Gabe, M. Calnan, and M. Bury. London: Routledge.

Farinella, D. 2005. *Privatizzazione e Cambiamento nel Servizio Pubblico*. Milano: FrancoAngeli.

Fedele, M. 1998. *Come Cambiamo le Amministrazioni Pubbliche*. Bari: Laterza.

Fennell, M.L. 1980. "The Effects of Environmental Characteristics on the Structure of Hospital Clusters." *Administrative Science Quarterly* 25: 484-510.

Ferrera, M. 2006. *Le Politiche Sociali. L'Italia in Prospettiva Comparata*. Bologna: Il Mulino.

Ferro, S., et al. 2008. *Assistenza All'ictus. Modelli Organizzativi Regionali*. Bologna: Agenzia Sanitaria Regionale.

France, G. 2008. "Seeking a Better Balance: Developments in Intergovernmental Relations in the Italian Health Care." *Eurohealth* 13 (3): 16-19.

France, G., and F. Taroni. 2005. "The Evolution of Health-Policy Making in Italy." *Journal of Health Politics, Policy and Law* 1-2: 169-184.

Freidson, E. 1970. *Profession of Medicine: A Study of the Sociology of Applied Knowledge*. New York: Harper & Row.

Gauld, R. 2001. "Contextual Pressures on Health. Implications for Policy Making and Service Provision." *Policy Studies* 22 (3-4): 167-179.

Glaser, B., and L. Strauss. 1967. *The Discovery of Grounded Theory*. Chicago: Aldine.

Granovetter, M. 1973. "The Strength of Weak Ties." *American Journal of Sociology* 78 (6): 1360-1380.

Granovetter, M. 2000. "Un'agenda Teorica per la Sociologia Economica." *Stato e Mercato* 60: 349-382.

Grol, R., and J. Grimshaw. 2003. "From Best Evidence to Best Practice: Effective Implementation of Change in Patients' Care." *Lancet* 362: 1225-1230.

Hatch, M.J. 1997. *Teoria Dell'Organizzazione*. Bologna: Il Mulino.

Hood, C. 1991. "A Public Management for All Seasons." *Public Administration* 69: 3-19.

Hood, C. 1995. "Emerging Issues in Public Administration." *Public Administration* 73: 165-183.

Jommi, C., and M. Del Vecchio. 2004. "I Sistemi di Finanziamento delle Aziende Sanitarie nel Servizio Sanitario Nazionale." *Mecosan* 49: 9-20.

Kazepov, Y., and A. Genova. 2005. "From Government Fragmentation to Local Governance: Welfare Reform and Lost Opportunities in Italy." In *Administering Welfare Reform: International Transformations in Welfare Governance*, eds. P. Henman, and M. Fenger. Bristol: Policy Press, 233-255.

King, G., R.O. Keohane, and S. Verba. 1994. *Designing Social Inquiry.* Princeton: Princeton University Press.

Krueger, R.A. 1994. *Focus Groups: A Practical Guide for Applied Research.* Thousand Oaks: Sage.

Langhorne, P., and M. Dennis. 2004. "Stroke Units: The Next 10 Years." *The Lancet* 363: 834-835.

Lanzalaco, L. 1995. *Istituzioni, Organizzazione, Potere.* Roma: NIS.

Lauria, G., M. Gentile, G. Fassetta, et al. 1995. "Incidence and Prognosis of Stroke in the Belluno Province, Italy. First-year Results of a Community-based Study." *Stroke* 26: 1787-1793.

Le Doare, K., D. Banerjee, and M. Oldfield. 2009. "Written Communication between General Practitioners and Hospitals: An Analysis." *West London Medical Journal* 1 (3): 67-75.

Liamputtong, P., and D. Ezzy. 2005. *Qualitative Research Methods.* Oxford: Oxford University Press.

Maarse, J.A.M., I.M. Mur-Veeman, and I.M.J.G Tijssen. 1990. "Changing Relations between Hospitals and Primary Health Care: New Challenges for Hospital Management." *International Journal of Health Planning and Management* 5 (1): 53-57.

Maino, F. 1999. "La Regionalizzazione della Sanità Italiana Negli Anni Novanta." *Il Politico* 4: 583-621.

Maino, F. 2001. *La politica sanitaria.* Bologna: Il Mulino.

Marshall, N. 1998. "How Well Do General Practitioners and Hospital Consultants Work Together? A Qualitative Study of Cooperation and Conflict within the Medical Profession." *British Journal of General Practice* 48 (432): 1379-1382.

Martelli, A. 2007. "Verso una Nuova Governance Locale delle Politiche Sociali?" *Autonomie Locali e Servizi Sociali* 1: 97-108.

Merton, R.K. 1949. *Social Theory and Social Structure.* New York: Free Press.

Nancarrow, S.A., and A.M. Borthwick. 2005. "Dynamic Professional Boundaries in the Healthcare Workforce." *Sociology of Health & Ilness* 27 (7): 897-919.

North, D.C. 1990. *Institutions, Institutional Change and Economic Performance.* Cambridge: Cambridge University Press.

Pavolini, E. 2009. "Is Regionalisation Good for your Health? The Experience of the Italian NHS." Paper presented at the *I Congreso Annual REPS, Oviedo.* http://www.espanet-spain.net/congreso2009/archivos/ponencias/TP09P04.pdf.

Pezzini, B. 2005. "Ventuno Modelli Sanitari? Quanta Disuguaglianza Possiamo Accettare (e Quanta Diseguaglianza Riusciamo a Vedere). Il Cosiddetto Modello Lombardo." In *I Servizi Sanitari Regionali tra Autonomia e Coerenze di Sistema*, ed. R. Balduzzi. Milano: Giuffrè, 399-424.

Putnam, R.D. 1993. *Making Democracy Work. Civic Traditions in Modern Italy.* Princeton: Princeton University Press.

Ranci, O.E. 2006. "Il Rapporto tra Servizi Sociali e Servizi Sanitari." In *La Riforma dei Servizi Sociali in Italia*, ed. C. Gori. Roma: Carocci, 116-127.

Ricci, S., M.G. Celani, F. La Rosa, et al. 1991. "SEPIVAC: A Community-Based

Study of Stroke Incidence in Umbria, Italy." *Journal of Neurology, Neurosurgery and Psychiatry* 54: 695-698.

Ross, A. 1967. *Directives and Norms*. New York: Humanity Press.

Rudd, A.G., A. Hoffman, P. Irwin, M. Pearson, and D. Lowe. 2005. "Stroke Units: Research and Reality. Results from the National Sentinel Audit of Stroke." *Quality and Safety in Health Care* 14 (1): 7-12.

Saka, O., V. Serra, Y. Samyshkin, A. McGuire, and C. Wolfe. 2009. "Cost-Effectiveness of Stroke Unit Care Followed by Early Supported Discharge." Stroke 40: 24-29.

Schein, E.H. 1985. *Organizational Culture and Leadership*. San Francisco: Jossey-Bass.

Sharpe, L.J. 1988. "The Growth and Decentralization of the Modern Democratic State." *European Journal of Political Research* 4: 365-380.

Simon, H. 1955. "A Behavioral Model of Rational Choice." *Quarterly Journal of Economics* 69: 99-118.

Sohn, M.W. 1997. "A Relational Approach to Measuring Competition among Hospitals." *Health Services Research* 37: 457-482.

Stivers, C. 2003. "Administration versus Management. Reading from Beyond the Boundaries." *Administration and Society* 35, 2: 210-230.

Stroke Unit Trialists' Collaboration. 2001. "Organised Inpatient (Stroke Unit) Care for Stroke." *Cochrane Database of Systematic Reviews* 3.

Taroni, F. 2007. "L'evoluzione delle Politiche Sanitarie in Italia, fra Crisi Finanziarie e Problemi di Fiducia." *Autonomie Locali e Servizi Sociali* 1: 29-42.

Trigilia, C. 1992. *Sviluppo Senza Autonomia*. Bologna: Il Mulino.

Vicarelli, G. 2005. "La Politica Sanitaria tra Obiettivi Annunciati e Effetti Inattesi." In *Il malessere del welfare*, ed. G. Vicarelli. Napoli: Liguori, 207-232.

Vicarelli, M.G., and E. Pavolini. 2009. "I Sistemi Sanitari Regionali in Italia: Trasformazioni e Rendimento in una Epoca di Regionalizzazione." In *Le Regioni. Capitale Sociale, Equilibri Politici e Rendimento Istituzionale*, ed. S. Vassallo. Bologna: Istituto Cattaneo.

Weick, K. 1969. *The Social Psychology of Organizing*. New York: McGraw Hill.

Do Local Government Units (LGUs) Interact Fiscally While Providing Public Health Services in the Philippines?

Uma Kelekar, *Marymount University*

Introduction

Historically, policymaking in developing countries has been highly centralized. These centralized systems emerged out of a strong colonial past or disenchantment with military rule or dictatorships (in the case of Latin America) in some of these countries (Asher, Newman, and Snyder 2002). In recent decades, however, decentralization has been at the center stage of policy experiments in many developing countries (Bardhan 2002, 1). Countries in Asia, Africa, and Latin America are increasingly involving lower tiers of government in delivery of public services that were earlier a responsibility of the central governments. Public services ranging from water, sanitation, education, and health are now provided by local governments in Uganda, the Philippines, Nigeria, and India. While local governments have limited revenue-raising capacity in developing countries as compared to the developed world, they enjoy substantial fiscal powers specifically in budgeting and spending.

To better understand the meaning of decentralization, a conceptual framework of four forms was developed, namely deconcentration, delegation, devolution, and privatization (Cheema and Rondinelli 1983). These forms differ in regard to the degree of discretion enjoyed by local bodies. A broad range of political, administrative, and fiscal responsibilities are transferred from the central government to regional, provincial, or municipal governments in decentralization. While deconcentration denotes transfer of administrative authority, delegation refers to transfer of authority over a specific set of tasks to local bodies such as state-owned enterprises. Devolution, on the other hand, is the transfer of authority to local governments that involves transfer of assets and rights, including fiscal powers of raising revenue and spending.

Health service decision making in developing countries like most public services was highly centralized with weak administrative capacity at the local government level (Mills et al. 1990). In the last few decades (1980s and 1990s) healthcare as a public responsibility has been devolved from national governments to sub-national governments in many developing countries.[1] The economic rationale for decentralization is mainly to allocate resources efficiently. Heterogeneous local needs are better satisfied by locally delivered services than when centrally provided. The reasons for devolving healthcare to local governments are similar. The theoretical arguments advanced for decentralizing healthcare are (a) increasing local ownership and accountability, (b) improving community participation, (c) strengthening integration of services at the local level, (d)

---

[1] An example of deconcentration is a district-level office of Ministry of Health where the lower-level offices are bestowed clearly defined functions, powers, or responsibilities by the higher-level government. The second form of decentralization is the delegation of government functions to private sector groups or non-government organizations who act as agents of the national government. Devolution is that wherein the LGUs are given full autonomy and control over assigned public services. Although they are overseen by the national government, they answer directly to the locally elected officials (Capuno 2009; Mills et al. 1990).

enhancing the streamlining of services and (e) promoting innovation and experimentation (Lakshminarayan 2003, 96).

On the other hand, a strand of public economics literature explores the possibility of fiscal interaction among jurisdictions in a decentralized system. There is some evidence of fiscal spillovers and strategic competition among devolved jurisdictions in providing health services in the context of developed countries (Costa-Font and Jordi Pons-Novell 2007; Moscone and Knapp 2005; Moscone, Knapp, and Tosetti 2007). However, there are a limited number of studies that examine the phenomenon for the developing world.

This paper therefore aims to fill this gap in the literature by examining fiscal spillovers in case of the Philippines. This paper is divided into five parts. First, the question of whether local governments in the Philippines interact fiscally with their neighbors is examined empirically with the help of 2007 health spending data. Preceding the empirical analyses, the first section discusses the relevant fiscal federalism literature including the concept of a public good, and provides an overview of the administrative and political structure of local governments in the Philippines. It also introduces the reader to the range of fiscal responsibilities of local governments specifically in the health sector after the country implemented its decentralization code in 1991. The first research question is derived in the second section, followed by a description of the model and methodology. The choice of variables is given in the third section. Descriptive statistics, regression results, and their interpretation are a part of the fourth section. In conclusion, the key empirical findings are reiterated along with some policy implications and future directions of research.

Literature Review

The term "pure public good" was first used by Samuelson (1954) to define collective consumption goods that people consume collectively such that an individual's consumption does not lead to a subtraction of the good for another individual's consumption. They are characterized as "non-rival" and "non-exclusive."[2] Samuelson (1958) however pointed out that not all goods provided by the government fall into this category of pure public goods. Buchanan (1965) filled this gap by defining "club goods" that share properties of "pure public goods" and "pure private goods." While one person may consume a pure private good at a point of time, not all public goods may be consumed by an infinite number of people such as police, parks, and fire services. The latter category of public goods is called "club goods."

Under microeconomic principles, healthcare may be classified as a public or private good based on its nature of consumption. Preventive health such as road safety and fluoridation of water, vaccinations, family planning, and health education are examples of public health goods. On the other hand, consumers draw exclusive benefits from privately consumed health services such as hospital care. Musgrave (1959) used the term merit goods to describe public health goods such as family planning, and immunizations as those whose private benefit is lesser than the social benefit. For instance, vaccination not only has direct benefits for persons inoculated but also accrues indirect benefits to non-

---

[2] A commonly used example of a public good is public defense provided to all citizens by the national government.

inoculated persons, as vaccinated people are less likely to transmit a disease (Boulier, Datta, and Goldfarb 2007).[3,4]

The theoretical background for this paper is drawn largely from the fiscal federalism literature that is related to the provision of publicly provided goods by local governments and its implications. While on the one hand, proponents of decentralization believe that local provision of public goods is the most efficient way of allocating resources and achieving societal welfare in an economy (Musgrave 1959; Oates 1972; Tiebout 1956). Proximity to local governments helps consumers reveal their true preferences by "voting with their feet," thus making the system more transparent and accountable (Tiebout 1956). Oates' decentralization theorem points to the appropriateness of a decentralized system:

[i]n the absence of cost-saving from centralized provision of a good and inter-jurisdictional externalities," he further states that *"the level of welfare will always be at least as high (and typically higher) if Pareto-efficient levels of consumption are provided in each jurisdiction than if any single, uniform level of consumption is maintained across all jurisdictions* (Oates 1972, 54).

Starett (1980) and Bewley (1981) illustrate non-Pareto states of equilibrium resulting from local provision of public goods in the presence of inter-jurisdictional spillovers and competition between regions. Local governments ignore social benefits of providing a public service in the presence of a spillover. Thus, due to the nature of non-excludability of local public goods (such as vaccinations), the marginal social benefit is higher than the marginal cost, leading local governments to under-supply the goods. Consistent with Olson (1971), although smaller jurisdictions might facilitate collective action among communities which encourages individuals to participate in local governance, localized decision making may give rise to inter-jurisdictional spillovers.

Fiscal interactions or competition among local governments have been a major area of theoretical work in public economics. Fiscal interactions among local governments take place in a number of situations (Zodrow and Mieszkowski 1986). First, regions may compete with each other in setting taxes and expenditures policies (Sinn 2003). For instance, in the *"race to the bottom,"* local officials may lower tax rates to attract more "businesses" and speed up economic development as compared to other regions. Second, fiscal interactions occur in the presence of spillovers. Second, fiscal interactions may also be induced by inter-jurisdictional competition among local political actors in the form of "yardstick competition." Residents of a region use their neighboring governments' performance as the yardstick to measure and evaluate the performance of their own government and whether they should seek to replace their governments in the next election period (Salmon 1987). Interdependence of fiscal policies at one level or more

---

[3] Boulier, Datta, and Goldfarb (2007), with the help of a susceptible-infectious-removed (SIR) model analytically present vaccination externalities and show marginal social benefits and externalities to vary with the number of vaccinations, vaccine efficacy, and infectiousness of the disease. As a higher number of people are vaccinated, non-inoculated persons continue to derive indirect benefits of not contracting the disease. Second, degree of externality may depend largely on the effectiveness of the vaccine and infectiousness of the disease. For instance, if vaccine efficacy is low, chances of inoculated people transmitting the disease are higher, driving the non-inoculated people to get vaccinated. The externality will thus be small. Third, if the disease is less infectious, the cost of inoculation may be perceived to be higher than the chances of contracting the disease. In this case, non-inoculated people will free ride on the inoculated people, increasing the extent of the externality (Boulier, Datta, and Goldfarb 2007).
[4] Musgrave used the term "merit wants" to signify "community wants or values" that individuals may wish to preserve even though they may conflict with individual preferences (Case 2008).

may result in distortions that prevent jurisdictions from achieving public sector equilibrium (Brueckner 1998). Third, fiscal inter-dependence in fiscal plans or competition among local governments might be the result of positive or negative spillovers that result from localized provision of public goods.

However, with respect to the health sector, the grounds for externalities are based on altruistic theories that support interdependence of utility functions between individuals (Hochman and Rodgers 1969). A great amount of theoretical evidence on altruism exists in the healthcare sector of developed countries. Hochman and Rodgers (1969) point to the importance of income redistribution in the form of fiscal transfers in order to achieve Pareto-efficiency.[5] And, therefore, spillovers of health benefits to neighboring regions arising from expenditures in a given region may not necessarily make its own residents worse off. This in turn may imply that in the presence of a positive spillover, a region may not necessarily adjust its spending.

Scholars provide a number of measures to mitigate the under-provision of public goods in the presence of spillovers. Central government intervention or forms of revenue sharing are a few recommendations made (Musgrave 1997; Oates 1999). Oates (1999), Tiebout (1956), and Williams (1966) recommend interaction and coordinated decision making between jurisdictions in order to minimize external economies and diseconomies. Contiguity facilitates integration of services and reduces diseconomies of scale, although not at the cost of reducing services or increasing costs. Coase (1960) emphasizes the importance of legal contracts or negotiations between parties in the presence of sufficiently low transaction costs, as a means to mitigate the divergence between private and social cost and achieve economic efficiency of resource allocation. Through compensation schemes between jurisdictions, Buchanan and Kaflogis (1963) and Williams (1966) show how local governments can achieve a socially optimal solution even in the presence of external economies.[6]

Several studies empirically test the presence of fiscal spillovers and policy inter-dependence among local governments in developed countries. Brueckner (1998) presents evidence of strategic interaction among cities of California in the imposition of growth control measures. Hanes (2002) provides evidence of fiscal interaction and under-provision of fire protection services among geographically contiguous Swedish municipalities. In a departure from the conventional definition of "geographical neighbors," Case, Rosen, and Hines (1993) investigate interdependence among jurisdictions that are similar with respect to income and demography instead of geographical proximity. People residing in states of similar demographic and economic characteristics are more likely to compete with each other in labor markets.

The negative effects of decentralizing public health services have been discussed widely in the literature (Kolehmainen-Aitken and Newbrander 1997). Decentralized health systems in the developed world that have recently been adopted by developing countries manifest externalities in the provision of public health services such as family planning, child and maternal health, and infant nutrition.

---

[5] Income differential and transfer elasticity of the donor were stated as vital in determining the desired amount of fiscal transfer (Hochman and Rodgers 1969).
[6] Buchanan and Kaflogis (1963) use the case of immunizations to show that when two parties yield external economies to each other, i.e., the externalities are reciprocal, cooperative purchase of the immunizations may lead to socially optimum position in which *fewer* immunizations are purchased than if each party acted independently. Thus, external economies need not result in an undersupply of aggregate resource inputs. Further, the output produced may be lower or higher than in the case of individual adjustment.

Khaleghian (2003) examine implications of political decentralized systems on the level of health services specifically immunizations among low- and middle-income countries and find significant differences between the two groups. While the impact of decentralization on immunization coverage is positive for low-income countries, it is on the other hand, negative for middle-income countries. The authors observed differences in the decentralization effect in low- and middle-income countries on account of different central–local relationships and patterns of community participation. Also, it was found that for a middle-income country like the Philippines, communities hold their public health officials responsible for curative spending as compared to preventive services due to the greater visible benefits associated with curative care.

The rationale for decentralization in developing countries is commonly justified on the basis of the "proximity principle" such as involvement of the local community in public decisions. Bardhan (2002) argues that the traditional fiscal federalism literature cannot be applied to decentralized systems in developing countries due to differences in their institutional design.[7] Therefore, local governments in developing countries are likely to behave in a different manner as compared to those in the developed countries due to differences in institutional (structure of incentives and organizations), administrative, and managerial and political factors.

Nevertheless, decentralized provision of health services in developing countries raises questions of whether local governments compete with each other in financing health services. Do local governments alter their public health expenditures positively or negatively in response to those of their neighbors? A few recent studies (Caldeira, Foucault, and Rota-Graziosi 2010; Arze del Granado, Martinez-Vasquez, and Simatupang 2008) discuss inter-jurisdictional competition in the context of developing countries. Arze del Granado, Martinez-Vasquez, and Simatupang (2008) explain fiscal competition in expenditures and taxes in Indonesia as a consequence of yardstick competition. Caldeira, Foucault, and Rota-Graziosi (2010) apply the fiscal federalism literature to Benin and identify fiscal interactions among *communes* that are geographically close to each other or with a similar ethnic structure. A positive and significant strategic interaction was found among communes, particularly in election periods.

Empirical studies on interdependence in health expenditures of local governments is however limited. Although a few studies (Moscone and Knapp 2005; Costa-Font and Jordi Pons-Novell 2007) investigate spatial dependence of health expenditures for developed countries, there is almost no similar work done for developing countries. Therefore, this paper aims to fill in this gap by using the Philippines, as a case study that has devolved significant responsibilities of public services to its local governments.

---

[7] For instance, the Tiebout hypothesis will not hold true in developing countries because people are not so mobile as to induce inter-jurisdictional competition among regions (Bardhan 2002).

Background

Geography, Politics, and Economy

The Philippines are a collection of 7,000 islands that are divided into three groups specifically Luzon, Visayas, and Mindanao. It is a middle-income country with a per capita Gross National Income of $3690 (for 2007 based on Purchasing Power Parity (PPP)) (World Bank). It is the world's 12th most populous country with a total population of 89 million comprising people from diverse cultures and ethnicities (NSO 2007). The country's population is predominantly young, with the 0–14 years age group representing 33.8 percent of the population while the elderly (over 65 years of age) make up about 4.4 percent of the total population (WHO).

The Philippines was under the authoritarian rule of Ferdinand Marcos from 1965 to 1986. At the end of the military rule, a new Constitution was ratified in 1987 that restored a pre-martial law constitutional system consisting of a President and Vice-President, bicameral legislature, and an independent Supreme Court. Political institutions in the Philippines are described as weak and political relationships as "clientelist" (Abinales and Amoroso 2005).

Administrative structure and fiscal responsibilities under the Local Government Code of 1991

The Philippines is divided into 15 administrative regions and 3 special regions namely Metropolitan Manila Development Authority (MMDA), Autonomous Region of Muslim Mindanao (ARMM), and Cordillera Administrative Region (CAR).[8] The nation-state is further divided into following the political sub-divisions (as of 2007):

- 80 provinces,
- 120 cities,
- 1511 municipalities, and
- 42,008 *barangays* or villages (NSCB, Philippines).

Under the Local Government Code of 1991 (LGC 1991), the creation of municipalities and cities was based on total income, population, and land area. Cities are classified into highly urbanized (33), independent component (5), and component cities (82). The highly urbanized areas and independent cities are independent of provinces. In addition, residents of independent component cities are prohibited from voting for provincial elective officials.[9] Component cities, on the other hand, are under the supervision of provinces in which they are geographically located (LGC 1991).[10]

Following decentralization, local government units (now onwards to be referred to as LGUs) assumed a key role in the delivery of public services such as health, education, agriculture, highway and public works maintenance and construction in the Philippines.

---

[8] In every regional capital, each of the 20 government departments have their regional offices.
[9] Residents of highly urbanized cities also remain excluded from the right to vote for elective provincial officials. However, qualified voters of cities who acquired the right to vote for elective provincial officials prior to the classification of cities as highly urbanized after the ratification of the Constitution and before the effectivity of the Code, shall continue to exercise such a right (Section 453, LGC 1991).
[10] If the component city is located within the boundaries of two or more provinces, it is considered a part of that province of which it used to be a municipality (LGC 1991).

The Local Government Code of 1991 stipulated broader taxing powers and increased the size of block grants namely internal revenue allotments (IRAs). Prior to devolution, 20 percent of the internally raised revenue was distributed to local governments. Under the new decentralization code, 40 percent of the revenue is distributed based on population (50 percent), land area (25 percent), and an equal share (25 percent). The aggregate IRA is divided among different local government levels as follows: 23 percent to provinces, 23 percent to cities, 34 percent to municipalities, and 20 percent to *barangays* (LGC 1991). The share is released directly to the provincial, city, municipal, or *barangay* treasurer.[11]

In addition to the internal revenue allotment, local government units (LGUs) receive a share of 40 percent of the gross collections from mining taxes, royalties, forestry and fishery charges, and other taxes, fees, and charges. They also receive a share from the proceeds of government agencies or government-owned or controlled organization. In addition, they receive a bulk of non-IRA funds in the form of discretionary allocations from national legislators called Priority Development Assistance Funds. The Code also allows LGUs to enter into contracts or inter-local agreements on grants, loans, and subsidies (LGC 1991) (for more details, see Appendix A).

The own-source revenue of LGUs comprises mainly taxes and user fees charged to residents, though some cities raise additional revenue by floating bonds, debentures, and securities in the market, under the vigilance of the Central Bank. As compared to municipalities, cities also stipulate taxes at a much higher rate. Additionally, LGUs exercise limited corporate powers of raising revenue by floating bonds in the private market (LGC 1991).[12]

On the expenditure side, local governments exercise almost complete discretion in utilizing its internal revenue allotment, after setting aside 20 percent as development fund (LGC 1991). The total LGU spending doubled from 1.6 percent of GDP in 1985–1991 to 3.5 percent in 1992–2007. Similarly, the average share of LGUs in government expenditure net of debt servicing rose from an average of 11.3 percent before LGC to an average of 24.2 percent in the post-LGC period (Manasan 2004).

From 1991 to 2007, the ratio of local government expenditure to GDP increased significantly for health spending. While the share of total health expenditure constitutes 3 percent of the country's GDP, the share of the local government aggregate expenditure on health rose from 0.08 percent in 1991 to 0.30 percent in 2007 (Manasan 2005).

The primary agents of public health spending in the Philippines are local government units (LGUs) that contribute to approximately 65 percent of the total spending. While the national government contributes its share of 13.19 percent, about 18.09 percent of the public health spending comes from foreign contributors and 4.20 percent from the rest of the world (National Health Accounts 2007). Local public health expenditure for cities and municipalities include expenditure on health programs such as medical, dental, health services, planning and administration of nutrition population, and family planning programs. The main components of public expenditure are:

•   personal services (PS) that include salaries and wages, personnel benefits contributions);

---

[11] The share is released on a quarterly basis within five days after the end of each quarter (LGC 1991).
[12] These should be revenue bonds whose proceeds shall be used to finance revenue-generating projects. Borrowing cannot exceed 20 percent of its own source revenue (LGC 1991).

- maintenance and other operating expenses (MOOE) covering supplies and materials, utility expenses, advertising, repairs and maintenance, communication, traveling and professional services; and
- capital outlays (National Health Accounts 2007).

As seen in Table 1, the central government retains monopoly power in enacting health legislation, setting regulations, and health standards, providing health education, and training medical personnel. It also provides personal care services in specialized tertiary-care hospitals managed by the Department of Health (DOH).[13] The provinces manage provincial health offices, provincial hospitals, and municipal and district hospitals that were previously managed by the central government. Provinces provide both primary and secondary health services.

Local governments including cities and municipalities provide primary healthcare services via primary health programs, maternal and child health, and communicable and non-communicable disease control services. They are responsible for procuring, storing and financing of drugs, medical supplies, and other equipment. Although vertical programs funded by international agencies are managed and controlled primarily by DOH, they are implemented with the help of municipalities and cities. However, there is some recent evidence of donor-funded maternal and child health programs being directly administered by LGUs (PIDS and UNICEF 2009).

Table 1. Functions of central government and local government units

	After devolution	Type of care
Central Government	Health policy, regulation and quality assurance, training and technical supervision, medical schools, and regional hospitals	Tertiary care
Local Government Units		
Provinces	Provincial/municipal or district hospitals	Primary/secondary care
Municipalities	Rural health units	Primary care/functions include delivery of maternal and child health programs, control of communicable diseases services, drug procurement, inventory, dispensing, and financing
Cities	City health offices/hospitals in highly urbanized cities	Primary care/secondary care
Barangays	*Barangay* health stations	Primary care

Source: Author compiled from different sources (Capuno 2009; Shwartz, Racelis, and Guilkey 2000; Shwartz, Guilkey, and Racelis 2002; Lakshminarayan 2003).

Decentralization that started almost two decades ago (in 1991) in the Philippines has yielded a significant improvement in the health and education outcomes. The progress in reducing infant and child mortality has been significant. Infant mortality rate dropped by 49 percent between 1990 and 2006. The under-five mortality rate also improved

---

[13] DOH has retained operation of 47 hospitals (National Capital Region hospitals, Special hospitals, Regional hospitals, and Specialty hospitals) and has added 20 more by reclassifying some provincial hospitals into regional or national centers (Shwartz, Racelis, and Guilkey 2000).

dramatically, falling by 53 percent from 1990 to 2006. Life expectancy at birth rose steadily from 66 in 1990 to 70 years in 2006 (Capuno 2009, 15).

Although the average gains in health outcomes might have been substantial, there are wide spatial variations across the country. Moreover, rising fertility and the high incidence of communicable and non-communicable diseases makes public health a challenging issue for its government.[14]

Research Design

Against the backdrop of the newly assigned responsibilities of local government units in the Philippines, this paper aims to identify any potential fiscal interactions in health spending for 2007. The year 2007 was selected for a number of reasons. The first and most important reason is that it is the latest year for which the fiscal, economic, demographic, and political variables data are readily available. Second, by 2007 decentralization in the Philippines was almost two decades old. This is presumably a long enough duration for the reforms to have been fully implemented and for any spillover effects to manifest.

The main research question is:

• *Are the changes in healthcare spending of a given region associated with the changes in the level of public health spending made by the neighbors?*

o *It is hypothesized that the health spending of local government units (in this case, municipalities/cities) is associated with that of the neighbors' health spending.*

The theoretical model used to answer the above research question is borrowed from the existing models based on maximization of indirect consumer utility in the presence of fiscal spillovers (Case, Rosen, and Hines 1994; Costa-Font and Jordi Pons-Novell 2007; Revelli 2003; Solé Olé 2005).

Following from Revelli (2003), assume that the society comprises two municipalities, i and j. An individual consumer's utility is a function of private and public goods consumed as well as individual tastes. In the presence of spillovers, consumer utility in municipality i is not only derived from public health services provided by its own government but also from those supplied in the neighboring municipality. Hence, consumer utility (u_i) is given as

$$u_i = f\{x_i, p_i, p_j, m_i\} \quad \text{Eq. (1)}$$

where x_i is the set of private composite goods, p_i the public health good supplied by its own municipality, p_j the public health good supplied by the neighboring municipality j, and m_i the other characteristics such as demographic structure, or individual preferences.

---

[14] The World Health Organization (WHO) classifies the Philippines as one of 22 high-burden countries, and ranks it eighth in the world in terms of estimated incidence of tuberculosis with 320 cases per 100,000 persons. Tuberculosis mortality in the Philippines is 54 per 100,000 persons. Due to its geographical location, the country faces various natural disasters such as typhoons, landslides, volcanic eruptions, and earthquakes (WHO).

On the other hand, individual consumers are constrained by their limited budget. Therefore, the total private consumption depends on total income (w_i), net of per capita tax (k_i), and contributions received from the government (g_i).

$$x_i = \{w_i - (k_i - g_i)\} \qquad \text{Eq. (2)}$$

The total public health good (p_i) supplied by municipality i is expressed as a function of the total population of the municipality (N_i) and per capita health expenditure (z_i).

In the presence of a horizontal interaction, p_i depends not only on the health expenditure of its own municipality but also on that of the neighboring municipality, where p_j is expressed as a function of total population (N_j) and per capita expenditure z_j. The parameter ρ measures the sign and magnitude of fiscal interaction between the two municipalities (Revelli 2003).

$$p_i = f\{(N_i * z_i),(N_j * z_j)^\rho\} \qquad \text{Eq. (3)}$$

The local government obtains the optimal per capita expenditure by maximizing the indirect utility function (the sum total of utilities of all the individuals in a society) (Eq. 4) subject to its own budget constraint (Eq. 5) as well as that of the consumers (Eq. 2).

$$W = \sum_{i=1}^{N} V\{f(x_i, p_i, p_j, m_i\} \qquad \text{Eq. (4)}$$

$$R = K + G + C \qquad \text{Eq. (5)}$$

where R is the total revenue, K the total tax revenue, G the inter-governmental grant, and C the all other receipts.

The total demand for the public health good (p_i) will depend on the public health good provided by the neighboring municipality (p_j), total residual income (x_i), implicit price of the public good (determined by per capita revenue, r_i) as well as individual characteristics (m_i) determined by the needs and preferences of the people (Eq. 6).

$$p_i = f(p_j, x_i, r_i, m_i\} \qquad \text{Eq. (6)}$$

Following from Revelli (2003), using Eqs. (3), (4), and (6), per capita health expenditure of municipality (z_i) (in log form) is determined (Eq. 7) as a function of the per capita health expenditure of the neighboring municipality (z_j), per capita income (x_i), grant size (g_i), total population (N_i), per capita revenue (r_i), and other economic, demographic, and political factors that might affect spending (m_i).

$$z_i = \rho \ln z_j + \beta \ln x_i + \beta \ln g_i, + \beta \ln N_i + \beta \ln r_i + \beta \ln m_i \qquad \text{Eq. (7)}$$

or

$$z_i = \rho \ln z_j + \beta_k \ln x_i + u_i \qquad \text{Eq. (8)}$$

where k is equal to the number of control variables.

The spatial lag model is theoretically consistent with a situation where regions interact with each other in determining their expenditure policies. (Brueckner 2003). The interdependency in fiscal policies of i and j municipalities in Eq. (8) is represented through a mixed regressive spatial autoregressive model, where the dependent variable per capita public health expenditure (z_i) of a region is a function of the weighted average expenditures of neighboring regions given by $\sum W_{ij} z_j$, where every neighbor receives an equal weight (Anselin 1988). The parameter ρ denotes the sign and magnitude of the interaction.

If an increase in expenditure of jurisdiction j (z_j) raises z_i, ρ will have a positive value, and the reaction function will be upward sloping. Conversely, if an increase in z_j decreases z_i, ρ will have a negative value and the reaction function will be downward sloping (Brueckner 2003).

$$z_i = \rho \sum W_{ij} z_j + \beta_k x_i + u_i; u \text{ f } N(0,1) \qquad \text{Eq. (9)}$$

A queen contiguity matrix is used to define neighborliness between local governments. The rationale behind the use of geographical distance is the nature of health as a good and the country's topography. In developing countries where transportation networks are not well developed, residents especially those located in more scattered islands of the Philippines have limited mobility. Unless they have to seek specialized curative care, they may not choose to travel long distances but rather seek access from immediate neighbors.

An additional complexity faced in the use of spatial econometric models is an endogenous dependent variable. Endogeneity refers to the simultaneity in the relationship between spatial neighbors. The expenditure of neighbor i affects the expenditure of neighbor j and expenditure of neighbor j also affects expenditure of i. This results in the dependent variable being correlated with the error terms. In order to obtain consistent estimates, a simultaneous estimation procedure is recommended such as instrumental variables (IV) or non-parametric maximum likelihood estimation (MLE) approaches.

Fiscal interactions in a decentralized system are well documented in the fiscal federalism and health economics literature. Therefore, the choice of a spatial autoregressive model with a spatially lagged dependent variable is justified based on economic theory and intuition in this analysis. Consistent with previous studies (Revelli 2003), a spatial lag model with an endogenous dependent variable is estimated using a two-stage least-squares estimation where the first stage involves identifying the relevant instruments. Anselin (1988) suggests the use of spatially lagged exogenous variables as appropriate instruments. Hence, the lagged exogenous variables here are used as instruments for the lagged per capita health expenditure.

Choice of Control Variables

Healthcare is a core component of human capital investment and critical for the economic progress of a country. Healthcare spending is associated with improved health outcomes, leading to higher workforce productivity and social welfare (Murthy and Okunade 2009).

The dependent variable in this analysis is per capita health expenditure. Traditionally, health expenditure has been studied as a function of economic, political, and demographic factors.[15] In addition, a few studies (Costa-Font and Jordi Pons-Novell 2007; Moscone and Knapp 2005; Moscone, Knapp, and Tosetti 2007) investigate the spatial component of expenditures.

Spatial interactions are highlighted as an important consideration in the empirical models of health expenditure determination among local governments, particularly for developed countries (Costa-Font and Jordi Pons-Novell 2007; Moscone and Knapp 2005; Moscone, Knapp, and Tosetti 2007). Biased results from exclusion of spatial dependence were confirmed in a few empirical studies.

In the context of health externalities, as discussed earlier, fiscal spillovers in financing public health are most likely to occur among local governments while providing maternal and child health services (like vaccinations and family planning) or control of infectious diseases (like malaria and dengue fever). Although the central government retains control of the provision of specific donor-funded preventive reproductive health programs such as family planning, local governments administer these vertical programs. Despite "Comprehensive Healthcare Agreements" set by the central government, it is not always the case that local governments comply with these provisions. Moreover, there is no punitive mechanism enacted against local governments that do not comply with these national standards. Second, there is evidence of local pressures (e.g., from the Catholic Church) that may not encourage the easy accessibility to certain controversial reproductive health services such as family planning (Lakshminarayan 2003).

Fiscal spillovers among governments may also arise in the provision of curative health services, specifically in the presence of cross-border utilization of medical services at hospitals run by provinces due to inter-provincial variations in quality of services (Capuno and Solon 1996). Within a system of competitive local governments, the latter may indirectly influence long-term decisions of people by discouraging patients with chronic care from settling in their jurisdictions by providing poor facilities or making access difficult. In addition, competition among provinces may occur if some provinces have their own insurance or health delivery programs.[16] Some of the innovative

---

[15] A few cross-country studies have attempted to study the relationship between technological progress and health care expenditure (Murthy and Okunade 2002; Di Matteo 2005).
[16] Bukidnon and Guimaras provinces have their own insurance programs. Some other cases include health card system of Paranaque city and Community Primary Hospital Program of Negros Oriental. Also, Malagag in

initiatives in health service delivery implemented by LGUs include charging graduated user fees to users based on their income levels or tapping external sources of funding to transform a rural health center into a community clinic. Besides benefiting its own residents, the community clinic in Sebaste serves residents of neighboring municipalities (Lieberman, Capuno, and Van Minh 2005).

Differences between regions with regard to the quality of health services provided might partly arise on account of drug procurement, inventory, dispensing, and financing systems of every LGU. This may translate into differences in quality, price, and supply of locally procured drugs and in turn determine the level of health service in the region (Lieberman, Capuno, and Van Minh 2005). While the case studies discussed suggest there may be a potential scope for negative fiscal interaction among LGUs, some empirical studies find evidence of positive fiscal interaction of healthcare expenditures in developed countries (Costa-Font and Jordi Pons-Novell 2007; Moscone and Knapp 2005; Moscone, Knapp, and Tosetti 2007). Studies that have found evidence of positive fiscal interaction of government expenditures in developing countries explain the phenomenon as a consequence of yardstick competition or strategic competition prior to an election period among political actors (Caldeira, Foucault, and Rota-Graziosi 2010). Ambiguity in the influence of fiscal interactions on per capita expenditures will be ruled out by empirically testing the hypothesis of whether or not local governments alter their health expenditure in response to their neighbors, and if so then in which direction?

Further, economists contend that income is an important determinant of total healthcare spending in a country (Newhouse 1977; Murthy and Okunade 2009; Parkin, McGuire, and Yule 1987). In conformity with the Wagnerian hypothesis that expenditures increase with an increase in income, several empirical studies re-confirm the positive influence of per capita income on per capita health expenditures of states and local regions (Case, Rosen, and Hines 1993; Costa-Font and Pons-Novell 2007; Di Matteo and Di Matteo 1998; Moscone, Knapp, and Tosetti 2007). Due to unavailability of data at the municipality level, provincial income per capita is used as a proxy for municipality or city income in the empirical analysis.

Total revenue per capita comprising own-source revenue and central government transfers is a fiscal variable used in the analysis. Based on theory, the influence of total revenue per capita is expected to be positive. Larger amounts of local resources at the disposal of an LGU are likely to drive a rise in per capita health spending. Similarly, higher per capita expenditures could be the result of larger grants received from the central government. Prior studies illustrate the influence of inter-governmental transfer payments on local government health expenditure in decentralized settings (Costa-Font and Pons-Novell 2007; Di Matteo and Di Matteo 1998).[17] Hence, this analysis also controls for the effect of IRA as a share of total revenue.

Population size tests for economies of scale incurred while providing healthcare services. Previous studies show a decline in per capita local government expenditure in response to rising population, indicating the presence of scale economies (Solé Olé 2005; Revelli 2003). Densely populated regions may also accrue scale economies. However, they may lead to congestion and hence demand higher per capita expenditures.

Davao del Sur and Sebaste in Antique started their own programs of health service delivery in their respective municipalities (Lieberman, Capuno, and Van Minh 2005).

[17] It is possible that local governments may strategically misrepresent their true needs and preferences in order to secure more than their fair share of resources from the central government.

Whether level of healthcare spending is commensurate with needs or preferences of the people is another question that is often raised in analyzing healthcare expenditures. A number of studies indicate that healthcare expenditure trends are associated with the aging of a population (Case, Rosen, and Hines 1993; Di Matteo and Di Matteo 1998). Further, certain segments of the population such as women and infants are more susceptible to communicable diseases, medical complications, and other illnesses. Healthcare expenditure, including medical or non-medical care expenditure, therefore may vary based on the age structure of the population.[18] A measure of demographic composition measured by percent of persons over the age of 60 is also controlled in one of the regression models. However, due to unavailability of data for all municipalities and cities, the percent of persons over 60 years is excluded from the spatial analyses.

Poverty is a complex phenomenon with many dimensions, including insufficient access to housing, food, nutrition, health, education, and leisure (Sen 1999). Traditionally, its statistical measure denotes the shortfall of income or consumption from a given threshold such as the poverty line. The measure of poverty incidence used in this study is defined as the proportion of people living in an area with an average per capita expenditure below the poverty line.[19],[20] Poorer regions associated with larger health needs but limited resources may either have a positive or negative relationship with health expenditures.

There are studies on political ideology impacting healthcare spending in the context of developed countries. Navarro and Shi (2001) and Navarro et al. (2006) contend that policies followed by social democratic and Christian democratic parties among OECD countries are aimed at reducing social inequalities and providing higher welfare and health services as compared to conservative parties.

Political parties in the Philippines are weak political structures and unable to perform efficiently as intermediate agents between state and society (Abinales and Amoroso 2005). Historically, small factions of elites, competing for the pool of resources from the central government, have dominated local politics in the Philippines. A distinct characteristic of Filipino political members is their shifting character of membership due to lack of ideological differences between parties. However, the church and religious groups play a dominant role in influencing the political decisions of the masses. The influence of church over policy issues such as family planning during Marcos-era, Aquino's, and Arroyo's presidencies is well documented. Arroyo cut the DOH budgets in 2003 for purchasing artificial contraceptives and announced support to the Catholic Church's natural family planning methods (Abinales and Amoroso 2005).

---

[18] In the year 2009, the distribution of limited swine flu vaccines in response to the outbreak of swine flu in the United States from the federal government to the states was based on the total size of states' population. The Center for Disease and Control of the United States, however, gave higher priority to more vulnerable sections of population such as pregnant women, people living with children younger than six months of age, healthcare and emergency medical services personnel, persons in the age group of six months and 24 years old, and persons over 24 with chronic health disorders or compromised immune systems. People over the age of 65 were not targeted because studies revealed that older populations were less vulnerable to the virus than the younger age group. (CDC, Questions and Answers, See link: http://www.cdc.gov/h1n1flu/vaccination/public/vaccination_qa_pub.htm).

[19] Logged average per capita household income and expenditure were predicted by combining survey data with auxiliary data obtained from Family Income and Expenditure and Labor Surveys, and the poverty measure was derived from them (Small-area Local Poverty Estimates 2005).

[20] Poverty line is estimated to represent monetary resources required to meet basic needs of members of households along with a non-food component (Small-area Local Poverty Estimates, NSCB 2005).

Patronage through discretionary funds that politicians seek is the most visible form of corruption in the government in the Philippines. An American politician used the quote *"All politics in the Philippines is local"* to describe the power of local politicians in the Philippines. The President, Vice-President, and Members of the Congress are elected with the help of a local network, often "[c]entered on the family and extended through their district by alliances and patronage" (Abinales and Amaroso 2005, 15). Congressional members from provincial districts nurture these networks through "pork-barrel funds" disbursed by the President.[21]

Political alliances between the President and the provincial governors have translated into benefits for the province due to reciprocity and granting of favors (personal and professional) between the two parties. For instance, in 2000 President Estrada conferred a higher share of tobacco excise tax to the Ilocos Sur governor, a crony of the latter in exchange for $8 million from illegal gambling (Abinales and Amoroso 2005). During election times, Presidential candidates rely on local politicians to garner local support.

Contrary to previous studies (Costa-Font and Pons-Novell 2007; Moscone, Knapp, and Tosetti 2007) that measure the influence of political parties' ideologies on healthcare spending, this paper does not consider political ideology as a control variable due to weak ideological affiliation of politicians to political parties. Instead, it attempts to capture the influence of pork barrel funding by including a dummy variable that measures whether the municipality or city mayor and their congressional district members belong to the same party. This political dummy variable is given a value of 1 if both politicians in the two administrative levels—municipality/city and congressional district belong to the same party, or 0 otherwise.[22][23]

The primary source of fiscal data is the Bureau of Local Government Finance. The remaining data on socioeconomic variables are obtained from several sources including the Bureau of Census and National Statistical Office, Philippines. Information on political parties is obtained from results published by the Commission of Elections (COMELEC) for the year 2004.

Regression Analysis

Table 2 presents the descriptive statistics of all variables used in the study. The average per capita revenue of municipalities is quite low as compared to cities. The IRAs make up a significant share of the total revenue of municipalities (84 percent), whereas at 61 percent it is much lesser for cities. Consistently, the average provincial per capita income of cities (PHP 29,582) is also higher than that of municipalities (PHP 22,992).

---

[21] A key characteristic of pre-modern Philippines' politics was concentration of power of local leaders called *datus*. The political community was defined by personal relationships maintained through networks of personal loyalties and marriages, and not territorial boundaries (Abinales and Amaroso 2005).

[22] Gloria Macapagal Arroyo was the elected President in the 2004 Presidential election and remained in office during the entire six-year period.

[23] Congressional members are elected from each district of a province. For example, if a province is a six congressional member district, and if four out of six candidates belong to Party LAKAS-CMD, then this province gets a value of LAKAS-CMD. If there is no clear majority of a party among congressional members then the province gets a value of "NO MAJORITY". The provincial value is matched against the mayor's party from every LGU. If there is a match, the dummy variable gets a value of 1. Otherwise, it gets a value of 0.

While the average per capita expenditure on health by a municipality is PHP 127, a city spends around PHP 185 Peso per capita. However, there are a few municipalities and cities in the National Capital Region that spend as high as PHP 1000 per capita.

Table 2. Descriptive statistics

Variables	Obs	Mean	Std. Dev.	Min	Max
Health expenditure pc					
Municipality	1,476	127	105	0	1,328
City	119	185	132	18	1,060
Total revenue pc					
Municipality	1,476	1,931	5,770	370	218,071
City	119	3,234	1,587	1,136	14,275
Provincial income					
Municipality	1,476	22,992	6,856	13,105	52,528
City	119	29,582	19,373	14,024	140,275
Percent of old					
Municipality	603	7.49	2.13	3.13	14.81
City	54	5.53	1.61	2.52	8.41

Figure 1 shows the geographic distribution of per capita health expenditures for LGUs. It is quite evident that expenditures tend to distribute in clusters with the highest concentration in the top-most Luzon region (high spending) and the southern-most Mindanao region (low spending). The Luzon region including the National Capital Region clearly spends much more on health per capita as compared to the Visayas (middle) and Mindanao regions.

The dataset for regressions excludes the stand-alone municipalities without any neighbors. Also, the observations with missing political data are excluded with their corresponding lagged observations. To induce normality, all variables are transformed into logarithmic forms and therefore the coefficients are to be interpreted as elasticities.

Model 1 presents OLS regression results of a sub-sample of 587 observations, for which data on elderly population was available. Share of elderly population as an independent variable was positively associated with health expenditures and was significant at 10 percent l.o.s.

As a first step, an OLS regression is run to identify any spatial dependence in error terms. The spatial statistics observed are Moran's I, Robust Lagrange Multiplier (LM) lag and error estimates. The Moran's I estimate is positive and significant, indicating a strong spatial positive autocorrelation of residuals.

The regression results, after correcting for endogeneity are listed under Model 3 in Table 3. After controlling for random provincial effects, ρ is positive and significant at 1 percent l.o.s.[24] The instruments used in the first-stage regression of the 2SLS estimation model are the lagged (first-order) independent variables affecting lagged per capita health expenditures.[25] The Anderson cannon LR and Hansen J statistics indicate that the instruments used in the first-stage regression of the two-stage least-squares estimation were appropriate and the model is identified.

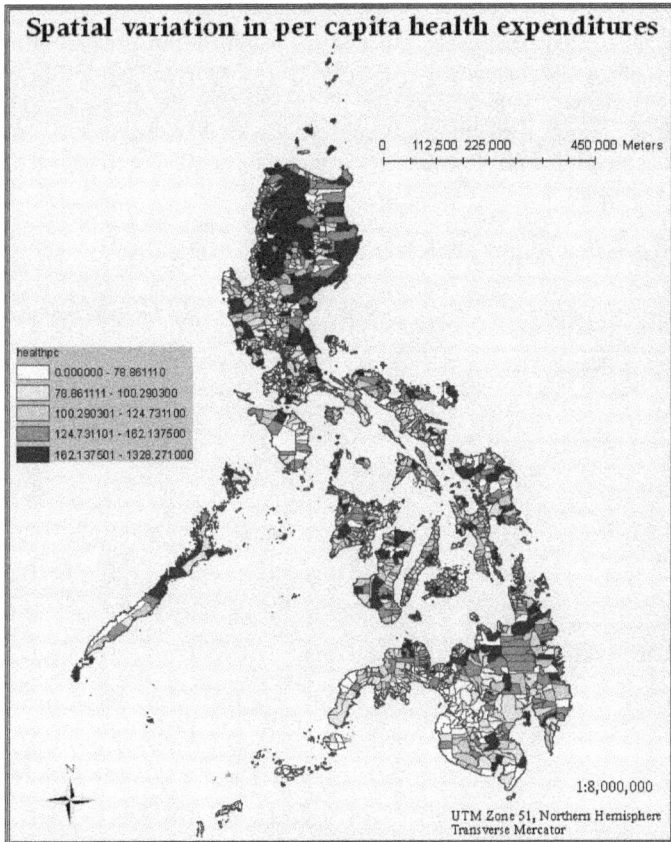

Figure 1. Spatial variation in per capita expenditures
Note: ARCGIS software was used to make the thematic maps.

---

[24] Spatial interaction was interacted with fiscal autonomy to test whether spatial interactions are higher among those LGUs with more fiscal autonomy. And there was no evidence in support of it.

[25] Second-order lagged independent variables were also used in addition to the first-order lagged variables as instruments. The instruments include lagged total revenue per capita, lagged political variable, lagged population, lagged population density, lagged IRA, lagged poverty incidence, and lagged provincial income. The reaction coefficient, although positive was marginally significant. This, however, may be attributed to the reduced sample size.

The signs were as expected for the remaining regressors.[26] A higher population is associated with lower per capita expenditures, implying the presence of economies of scale.[27] Population density is negative and insignificant. All the fiscal variables have a positive and significant impact on per capita health expenditures. Poverty incidence is negatively associated with expenditure while provincial income influences expenditures positively. The political variable that measures the pork-barrel effect is positive and significant. This may imply that political actors, at the local and national levels may influence the availability and use of funds.

A strong and positive spatial dependence on public health expenditures is a key finding of this study. An increase of one percent of neighboring local government expenditure is associated with an increase of 0.1053 percent in the level of health spending of a given region. This finding is consistent with the previous studies on spatial dependence in general public expenditures among local governments in developing countries such as Indonesia and Benin.

Table 3. Regression results of horizontal fiscal interaction

Dependent/independent variable	Model 1 (OLS)	Model 2 (OLS)	Model 3 (2SLS)
Dependent variable: health expenditure per capita			
Provincial income	0.2264***	0.1559***	0.1825***
	(0.0651)	(0.0570)	(0.0613)
Poverty incidence	−0.0265	−0.0362	−0.0636*
	(0.0397)	(0.0311)	(0.0353)
Population	−0.1586***	−0.03412*	−0.0499***
	(0.0684)	(0.0175)	(0.0181)
Population density	−0.0296	−0.0046	−0.0195
	(0.0294)	(0.0178)	(0.0202)
Total revenue pc	0.7488***	0.6745***	0.7132***
	(0.0512)	(0.0541)	(0.0506)
Share of IRA in total revenue	0.2481***	0.2174***	0.2228***
	(0.0856)	(0.0585)	(0.0591)
Political dummy	0.0712***	0.0810***	0.0876***
	(0.0221)	(0.0206)	(0.0219)
ρ	0.0995**	0.2672***	0.1053**
	(0.0412)	(0.0575)	(0.0464)
Percent of Old	0.1512*		
	(0.0843)		
Province effects clustered	Yes	Yes	Yes
Sample size	587	1363	1363
R^2	0.6267	0.5091	0.4983
Anderson canon LR statistic			776.678***
Hansen J statistic			5.688
			(0.4591)

---

[26] Although some of the control variables (such as total revenue per capita) are endogenous in the model presented in the second section, they are treated as exogenous in the empirical specification.
[27] An alternative explanation for the negative coefficient of population could be that the revenues do rise commensurate with population or fiscal need, thus indicative of a fiscal gap (Manasan 1998).

Notes: The lagged control variables were the instruments used in the first-stage regression.
Model 3 includes first-order lagged instruments.
The figures in parenthesis are the robust standard errors of the coefficients.
The province-level common shocks are controlled in each of the models.
The spatial lags as well as spatial statistics were estimated using the GEODA software.
Province-level fiscal interactions were also examined. Consistent with theory, there was no significant interaction observed at that level.
*, **, *** indicate levels of significance at 10, 5, and 1 percent level of significance (l.o.s).

Several explanations can be given to justify the above result.[28] One potential cause of positive spatial dependence is bidding by municipalities for medical supplies such as drugs and specialized personnel like doctors. Competition between municipalities drives cost of health inputs to rise and induces strategic interaction in spending.

Municipalities in the Philippines are responsible for procuring, storing, and financing their drugs and other medical supplies. Lieberman, Capuno, and Van Minh (2005, 15) discuss the corrupt bidding practices prevalent in the local drug procurement system. "Bids are rigged, qualified bidders are pre-identified, and bidders connive."[29] This causes stock shortages, poor quality of drugs and purchase prices to be much higher than private pharmacies.

They also point out the difficulties faced by local governments in hiring physicians, nurses, and medical technicians that are in great demand in foreign markets. Further, local governments may be compelled to out-perform other LGUs by attracting physicians with offers such as "attractive salaries, honoraria such as free board and lodging." Under the decentralized system, despite the salary guidelines prescribed by the Civil Service Commission, local governments are given some autonomy in determining compensation for their employees. Differentiation in rates of pay among LGUs arises on account of different income classes and different levels of administration (Manasan and Castel 2010). First, there is a different salary grade assigned to the same position in LGUs depending on whether it is in a province, city, or municipality. The second level of differentiation is based on the income class of the LGU. Non-uniformity in the salaries and benefits offered to doctors in LGUs of different incomes and levels indicate that this might be one of the potential causes of spatial competition of health spending (see Figure 2).

---

[28] Another explanation offered might be based on altruistic theories where the overall health outputs produced in the presence of negative spillovers may be optimal due to the nature of health externalities. An improvement in health outcomes of neighboring governments (that may be caused by higher health spending in a given region) does not necessarily make residents of a given region worse off. Despite the possibility of free riding by neighboring regions a given region may not reduce its health spending.

[29] Local governments in decentralized systems seek their estimated supply of vaccines, transportation, and other supplies from the central governments that in turn allow local health providers to bid for the vaccines and other supplies.

Compensation of doctors in the LGUs

Based on the fiscal capacity of the LGUs and guidelines set by the Department of Budget and Management (DBM), the legislative bodies are able to provide additional allowances and benefits to the health officials. The flexibility enjoyed by LGUs in determining wages increased with the passage of the Senate and House Representatives Joint Resolution No. 1 in 1994, thus allowing LGUs (except special cities and first class cities) to adopt one out of the eight salary schedules of higher class LGUs subject to certain conditions (Manasan and Castel 2010).

Originally, the LGC limited spending of LGUs belonging to income class 1–3 and those belonging to 4–6 classes to 45 and 55 percent on personnel services (PS) respectively. Due to difficulty faced by LGUs in adhering to the PS cap, the Department of Budget and Management introduced "waivers" excluding items such as Magna Carta for Public Health Workers. Under the Magna Carta Benefits for Public Health Workers (Republic Act 7305), health workers are granted subsistence allowance, laundry allowance, night-shift differential, hazard pay, and longevity pay (Manasan and Castel 2010).

Figure 2. Compensation of doctors in the LGUs

Positive fiscal interactions, as discussed in the literature, may also be on account of yardstick competition between local governments. However, existence of yardstick competition is debatable in young democracies such as the Philippines (Caldeira, Foucault, and Rota-Graziosi 2010). Caldeira, Foucault, and Rota-Graziosi (2010) find evidence of opportunistic behavior among local governments in the form of positive fiscal interactions, especially during election time.

Drawing from their findings, one of the possible reasons for spatial dependence in the Philippines could be that the given year of analysis (i.e., 2007) was an election year for local governments. So in order to be re-elected to public office, it is possible that in that year they strategically competed with each other by providing higher public health services to its residents as compared to its neighbors.

Policy Implications and Conclusions

Fiscal decentralization has been a part of many public sector reforms in the developing world. This paper examines the implications of decentralization on health spending. The main purpose is to test for fiscal spillovers and interactions among local government units (LGUs) (including municipalities and cities) in the Philippines using health expenditure data for the year 2007.

Fiscal decentralization in the Philippines is perceived to have facilitated the improvement of health outcomes in the long run. While there is concern raised with respect to the increased health spending in the post-devolution era, some experts believed that decentralization mitigated the high costs borne by the central government in facilitating travel to different islands prior to devolution.

One of the advantages of decentralization in developing countries, as supported by some case studies in the Philippines is the role of the local communities in public decisions (Lieberman, Capuno, and Van Minh 2005). However, some scholars have stressed that due to institutional differences between the developing and the developed countries, traditional fiscal federalism theory, which has primarily developed in the context of developed countries may not be relevant to other developing countries. For instance, people in the developing countries may not be very mobile and hence would not be expected to "vote with their feet." The efficiency argument in favor of decentralization in the developing countries is consequently weak. This paper provides empirical evidence of fiscal interactions among LGUs, a result of decentralized provision of health services. Within a spatial econometrics framework, spatial lag models are used to estimate spatial dependence on health expenditures among LGUs. Neighbors are determined with the help of a contiguity-based (queen contiguity) matrix.

This paper aims to answer one main research question. It tests for horizontal fiscal interactions in health spending among municipalities. One of the key findings of this paper is a strong and positive spatial dependence on health expenditures among LGUs. On average, an increase of one percent of neighboring local government expenditure is associated with an increase of 0.1073 percent in the level of health spending of a given region. The findings of this analysis have been consistent with earlier studies investigating fiscal spillovers in health expenditures. However, the reasons given to explain this phenomenon are placed in the context of the Philippines' politics and institutions. The spatial interaction in health expenditures among LGUs has been explained as an outcome of competition driven by constraints in resources and infrastructure. One of the potential explanations is the limited supply of resources such as doctors that might be causing LGUs to compete for personnel by outperforming the benefits' packages offered by its neighboring LGUs. Differentiation in the salaries of doctors across the LGUs has been discussed as a potential source of competition.

Another possible explanation given for the positive fiscal interaction of health is that of strategic competition among political actors. Yardstick competition has been debatable in the context of the developing countries to explain positive spatial dependence on public spending.[30] However, there are studies that indicate that positive spatial dependence on health spending might be a part of a political agenda. Political actors might wish to strategically out-spend their neighbors in order to get re-elected to public office. Political competition has been one of the reasons given to explain the positive spatial dependence in health spending, considering that the year of the analysis, i.e., 2007 was an election year.

As a future direction of research, the analysis will be carried out for a panel dataset comprising a longer duration including both, election and non-election years in order to test the validity of political competition as an explanation of horizontal fiscal interaction. Second, the analysis relied on spatial lag models for all the empirical analyses. Although the standard errors take into account random provincial effects, it might be helpful to test the robustness of the empirical results by using variations of spatial models that incorporate a spatially autoregressive disturbance term. Third, it would be interesting to test the robustness of the empirical findings by using some other matrices to define neighborliness. The current contiguity matrix excludes the possibility of interactions

---

[30] Yardstick competition is where residents of a region use their neighboring governments' performance as the yardstick to measure and evaluate the performance of their own government and whether they should seek to replace their governments in the next election period (Salmon 1987).

between landmasses. Therefore, testing for such interactions could be accomplished through the use of distance-based matrices and comparing the results to the adjacency-based matrices. However, arguably the use of the contiguity based matrices makes the empirical results of this paper relevant to other contiguously developing countries.

This paper aims to draw the attention of policymakers to several issues.

Inequitable access to resources: It is consistent with the quantitative analysis and expert interviews where some LGUs have an advantage over others in access to resources. This in turn may result in disparities in the level of health services provided by the LGUs. Therefore, a more uniform distribution of public services may require granting low-income class LGUs the ability to raise additional revenue and develop their infrastructure.

Past literature indicates that due to inefficiencies in the use of funds and low level of trust in the local governments, people are not willing to pay higher local taxes that in turn restrict the local governments from upgrading their services without relying on central government funds. There have been recommendations made in the House and Senate about revisiting the formula for allocating IRAs and incorporating factors of fiscal capacity and/or needs of regions to ensure a more efficient use of transfers (Llanto 2009).

Need to conduct regular audits: It may also be useful to develop an entity to monitor the use of local and national government funds. Regular audits held by independent investigating bodies prior to local and national elections might be necessary to prevent unnecessary politically motivated spending.

Inter-jurisdictional cooperation through Inter-Local Health Zones: Although the Local Government Code (LGC) specifies Inter-Local Health Zones as a means to promote inter-jurisdictional cooperation to facilitate coordination of resources, they are limited in their effectiveness. The central government might have to take some proactive steps to encourage inter-jurisdictional co-ordination through inter-local health zones.

Integration of labor markets: Finally, a proper integration of labor markets as well as revisiting the payment structure for health workers by the central government might be a necessary step in reducing competition among LGUs for scarce resources such as doctors.

Appendix A
Table A1. Classification of revenue of local government units

GENERAL FUND			
TAX REVENUE	*Provincial/city impositions* Real property tax • Basic tax** • Special levy ** Proceeds are distributed between cities, municipalities and *barangays* within the Metropolitan Manila Area (Section 271).	Tax on business *Provincial/city impositions* • Business of printing and publications • Franchise tax • Tax on sand, gravel, and quarry resources* • Amusement tax on admission • Tax on amusement places* • Annual fixed truck on delivery trucks or vans * Municipalities/*barangays* have shares in the proceeds	Other taxes *Provincial/city impositions* • Tax on transfer of real property ownership* • Professional tax • Other impositions
		City/municipal impositions • Manufacturers, assemblers • Wholesalers, distributors • Exporters or manufacturers, dealers of essential commodities • Retailers • Contractors and other independent contractors • Banks and other financial institutions • On peddlers • Other business taxes	*City/municipal impositions* • Community tax • Other impositions
NON-TAX REVENUE	Regulatory fees • Mayor's permit • Permit fees under the building code • Zonal/locational clearance fees • Fees on weights and measures • Motorized tricycle operator's permit • Cattle registration fees • Civil registration fees • Slaughter permit fee • Other regulatory fees • Toll fees	Service/user charges • Secretary's fees • Garbage collection fees • Parking fees • Other receipt/user charges (sanitary inspection fees, health examination fees) Other receipts • Fishery rentals • Sales of assets • Miscellaneous receipts	Receipt from Economic Enterprises • Receipts from markets • Receipts from slaughter houses • Receipts from cemeteries • Receipts from bus terminals • Rentals • Receipts from waterworks systems • Other receipts from economic enterprises

SHARES FROM NATIONAL TAX	National tax collections • Internal Revenue Allotment (IRA) • Local Government Stabilization and Equalization Fund (LGSEF) • Local Affirmative Action Project Fund (LAAPF) • Priority Development Assistance Fund (PDAF)*** • Share in National Wealth • Share in Tobacco Excise Tax • Share in Expanded Value-added tax • Share from Economic Zones *** Allocated to Congress members for discretionary spending in LGUs.	Extraordinary receipts/grants/aids • Grants^—foreign and domestic 1. Calamity Fund 2. Municipal Development Fund 3. Local Government Empowerment Fund 4. Countryside Development Fund 5. DECS School Building Program • National Aids • Share from Lotto • Rebates on MMDA Contributions • Other extraordinary receipts ^Conditional cash grants are given to extremely poor households a Poverty reduction and social development program called Pantawid Pamilyang Pilipino Program (4Ps).	Loans and borrowing • Foreign • Domestic • Bond floatation
SHARES FROM NATIONAL TAX	Inter-local transfers		

Source: Local Government Code 1991.

166

References

Abinales, Patricio N., and Donna J. Amoroso. 2005. *State and Society in the Philippines*. Lanham, MD: Rowman and Littlefield Publishers, Inc

Anselin. 1988. *Spatial Econometrics: Methods and Models. Studies in Operational Regional Science*. Dordrecht, The Netherlands: Kluwer Academic Publishers.

Arze del Granado, J., J. Martinez-Vazquez, and R.R. Simatupang. 2008. "Local Government Fiscal Competition in Developing Countries: The Case of Indonesia." *Urban Public Economic Review* 008: 13-45.

Asher, Mukul G., David Newman, and Thomas P. Snyder. 2002. *Public Policy in Asia: Implications for Business and Politics*. West Port, CT: Quorum Books.

Bardhan, Pranab. 2002. "Decentralization of Governance and Development." *Journal of Economic Perspectives* 16 (4): 185-205.

Bewley Truman, F. 1981. "A Critique of Tiebout's Theory of Local Public Expenditures." *Econometrica* 49 (3): 713-740.

Boulier, Bryan L., Tejwant S. Datta, and Robert S. Goldfarb. 2007. "Vaccination Externalities." *The B.E. Journal of Economic Policy and Analysis* 7 (1), Article 23: 1-25.

Brueckner, Jan K. 1998. "Testing for Strategic Interaction among Local Governments: The Case of Growth Controls." *Journal of Urban Economics* 44 (3): 438-467.

Brueckner, Jan K. 2003. "Strategic Interaction Among Governments: An Overview of Empirical Studies." *International Regional Science Review* 26 (2): 175-188.

Buchanan, James M. 1965. "An Economic Theory of Clubs." *Economica* 32: 1-14.

Buchanan, James M., and Milton Z. Kafoglis. 1963. "A Note on Public Goods Supply." *The American Economic Review* 53 (3): 403-414.

Bureau of Local Government Finance. Philippines: Department of Finance.

Caldeira, Emilie, Martial Foucault, and Gregoire Rota-Graziosi. 2010. "Decentralization in Africa and Fiscal Competition: Evidence from Benin." *Scientific Series*, CIRANO, Quebec, Montreal.

Capuno, Joseph J. 2009. "A Case of Decentralization of Health and Education Services in the Philippines." HDN Discussion Paper Series, PHDR Issue 2008-2009, No. 3.

Capuno, Joseph J., and Orville C. Solon. 1996. "The Impact of Devolution on Local Health Expenditures: Anecdotes and Some Estimates from the Philippines." *Philippine Review of Economics and Business* 33 (2): 283-318.

Case, Karl E. 2008. "Musgrave's Vision of the Public Sector: The Complex Relationship Between Individual, Society and State in Public Good Theory." *Journal of Economic Finance* 32 (July): 348-355.

Case, Anne C., Harvey S. Rosen, and James C. Hines. 1993. "Budget Spillovers and Fiscal Policy Interdependence." *Journal of Public Economics* 52 (3): 285-307.

Center for Disease and Control (CDC). Questions and Answers. http://www.cdc.gov/h1n1flu/vaccination/public/vaccination_qa_pub.htm.

Cheema, G. Shabbir, and Dennis A. Rondinelli, eds. 1983. *Decentralization and Development: Policy Implementation in Developing Countries*. Beverly Hills, CA: Sage Publications.

Coase, Ronald H. 1960. "The Problem of Social Cost." *Journal of Law and Economics* 3: 1-44.

Costa-Font J., and Jordi Pons-Novell. 2007. "Public Health Expenditure and Spatial Interactions in a Decentralized National Health System." *Health Economics* 16 (3): 291-306.

Hanes, Niklas. 2002. "Spatial Spillover Effects in the Swedish Local Rescue Services." *Regional Studies* 36 (5): 531-539.

Hochman, Harold M., and James D. Rodgers. 1969. "Pareto Optimal Redistribution." *American Economic Review* 59 (4): 542-557.

Khaleghian, Peyvand. 2003. "Decentralization and Public Services: The Case of Immunization." Policy Research Working Paper 2989, World Bank.

Kolehmainen-Aitke, Riitta-Liisa, and William Newbrander. 1997. *Decentralizing the Management of Health and Family Planning Programmes.* Boston, MA: Management Sciences for Health. Processed.

Lakshminarayan, Rama. 2003. "Decentralization and its Implications for Reproductive Health: The Philippines Experience." *Reproductive Health Matters* 11 (21): 96-107.

Lieberman, Samuel S., Joseph J. Capuno, and Hoang Van Minh. 2005. "Decentralizing Health: Lessons from Indonesia, The Philippines and Vietnam." *East Asia Decentralizes: Making Local Governments Work.* Washington DC: The International Bank for Reconstruction and Development/ The World Bank Publication.

Llanto, Gilbert M. 2009. "Fiscal Decentralization and Local Finance Reforms in the Philippines." Discussion Paper Series No. 2009-10, Philippines Institute for Development Studies.

Manasan, Rosario G. 2004. *Local Public Finance in the Philippines: Balancing Autonomy and Accountability.* Philippines: Philippines Institute for Development Studies.

Manasan, Rosario G. 2005. "Local Public Finance in the Philippines: Lessons in Autonomy and Accountability." *Philippine Journal of Development* 32(2): 31-101.

Manasan, Rosario G., and Cynthia G. Castel. 2010. "Study of Local Personal Services Expenditure Policy." In *Fiscal Decentralization in the Philippines: Issues, Findings and New Directions*, eds. Tariq H. Niazi, Gilbert Llanto, and Raymund Fabre. Philippines: Department of the Interior and Local Government and Asian Development Bank.

Di Matteo, Livio. 2005. "The Macro Determinants of Health Expenditure in the United States and Canada: Assessing the Impact of Income, Age Distribution and Time." *Health Policy* 71: 23-42.

Di Matteo, Livio and Rosanna Di Matteo. 1998. "Evidence on the Determinants of Canadian Provincial Government Health Expenditures: 1965–1991." *Journal of Health Economics* 17: 211-228.

Mills, Anne, et al., eds. 1990. *Health System Decentralization: Concepts, Issues and Country Experiences.* England: World Health Organization.

Moscone, Francesco, and Martin Knapp. 2005. "Exploring the Spatial Pattern of Mental Health Expenditures." *The Journal of Mental Health Policy and Economics* 8: 205-217.

Moscone, Francesco, Martin Knapp, and Elissa Tosetti. 2007. "Mental Health Expenditure in England: A Spatial Panel Approach." *Journal of Health Economics* 26: 842-864.

Murthy, Vasudeva N.R., and Albert A. Okunade. 2009. "The Core Determinants of Health Expenditures in the African Context: Some Econometric Evidence for Policy." *Health Policy* 91: 57-62.

Musgrave, Richard. 1959. *The Theory of Public Finance: A Study in Public Economy*. New York: McGraw Hill.

Musgrave, Richard. 1997. "Reconsidering the Fiscal Role of Government." *The American Economic Review* 87 (2): 156-159.

National Health Accounts (NHA). 2007. National Statistical Organization, Philippines. National Statistical Co-ordination Board (NSCB). http://www.nscb.gov.ph/.

National Statistical Coordination Board. 2005. "Estimation of Local Poverty in the Philippines." National Statistics Office (NSO), Republic of the Philippines. http://www.census.gov.ph/.

Navarro, Vicente, and Leiye Shi. 2001. "The Political Context of Social Inequalities and Health." *Social Science and Medicine* 52: 481-491.

Navarro, Vicente et al. 2006. "Politics and Health Outcomes." *Lancet* 368: 1033-1037.

Newhouse, Joseph P. 1977. "Medical Care Expenditure: A Cross-national Survey." *The Journal of Human Resources* 12 (1): 115-125.

Oates, Wallace E. 1972. *Fiscal Federalism*. New York: Harcourt Brace Jovanovich.

Oates, Wallace. 1999. "An Essay on Fiscal Federalism." *Journal of Economic Literature* 37: 1120-1149.

Olson, Mancur. 1971. *The Logic of Collective Action: Public Goods and the Theory of Goods*. USA: Harvard University Press.

Parkin, David, Alistair McGuire, and Brian Yule. 1987. "Aggregate Health Care Expenditures and National Income: Is Healthcare a Luxury Good?" *Journal of Health Economics* 6 (2): 109-127.

National Statistics Office (NSO) (2007). Philippines. http://www.census.gov.ph/.

Philippine Institute for Development Studies and the United Nations Children's Fund (UNICEF). 2009. "Improving Local Service Delivery for the MDGs in Asia: The Case of the Philippines." Discussion Paper Series No. 2009-34.

Republic of the Philippines Congress. Republic Act No. 7160. 1991. "An Act Providing For A Local Government Code of 1991".

Revelli, Frederico. 2003. "Reaction or Interaction? Spatial Process Identification in Multi-tiered Government Structures." *Journal of Urban Economics* 53 (1): 29-53.

Salmon, Pierre. 1987. "Decentralisation as an Incentive Scheme." *Oxford Review of Economic Policy* 3 (2): 24-43.

Samuelson, Paul. 1954. "The Pure Theory of Public Expenditures." *The Review of Economics and Statistics* 36 (4): 387-389.

Samuelson, Paul. 1958. "Aspects of Public Expenditure Theories." *The Review of Economics and Statistics* 40 (4): 332-338.

Sen, Amartya K. 1999. *Commodities and Capabilities*. USA: Oxford University Press.

Shwartz, J. Brad, Rachel Racelis, and David K. Guilkey. 2000. "Decentralization, and Local Government Health Expenditures in the Philippines." Measure Evaluation Project, Working Paper 01-36.

Shwartz, J. Brad, David K. Guilkey, and Rachel Racelis. 2002. "Decentralization, Allocative Efficiency and Health Service Outcomes in the Philippines." Measure Evaluation Project, Working Paper 02-44.

Sinn, Hans-Werner. 2003. *The New Systems Competition*. Oxford: Wiley Blackwell Publishing.

Solé Ollé, Albert. 2005. "Expenditure Spillovers and Fiscal Interactions: Empirical Evidence from Local Governments in Spain." *Journal of Urban Economics* 59 (1): 32-53.

Starett, David A. 1980. "Measuring Externalities and Second Best Distortions in the theory of Local Public Goods." *Econometrica* 48 (3): 627-642.

Tiebout, Charles. 1956. "A Pure Theory of Local Expenditures." *The Journal of Political Economy* 64 (5): 416-424.

Williams, Alan. 1966. "The Optimal Provision of Public Goods in a System of Local Government." *Journal of Political Economy* 74 (1): 18-33.

World Bank. "World Development Indicators." International Comparison Program Database. http://data.worldbank.org/indicator/NY.GNP.PCAP.PP.CD.

World Health Organization (WHO), Philippines. http://www.wpro.who.int/countries/phl/en/.

Zodrow, George R., and Peter Mieszkowski. 1986. "Pigou, Tiebout, Property Taxation and Under-provision of Local Public Goods." *Journal of Urban Economics* 19: 356-370.

IV. Political Theory and Practice

Stem Cells, Cloning, and Political Liberalism

Bonnie Stabile, *George Mason University*

Purpose

This chapter proposes to examine the policy predicament posed by human embryonic stem cell research and cloning through the lens of political liberalism to consider how such controversies can be reasonably resolved in a constitutional democracy. Stem cell research, because of its use of human embryos and the potential for human cloning, is one of the most complex and controversial issues of our time. Governments crafting stem cell policies find the process confounded both by the complexity of the science involved and by the panoply of deeply felt moral and ethical responses it has provoked. The conundrum is characterized by polarized political views and personal opinions running the gamut from confused to dogmatic. In the face of such intractable and divisive social controversies, citizens sometimes wonder how the convictions of those on different sides of the aisle can ever be reconciled to create policies palatable to both, and whether the virulent debates of those with starkly opposing views threaten to tear at the fabric of social concord.

John Rawls suggests that, "we turn to political philosophy when our shared political understandings ... break down, and equally when we are torn within ourselves" (44). In the face of particularly thorny political problems, a return to relevant philosophical roots suggests a framework for understanding how diverse views are contained or accommodated in a constitutional democracy. Political liberalism tries to answer the very question that concerns us: "how is it possible that there can be a stable and just society whose free and equal citizens are deeply divided by conflicting and even incommensurable religious, philosophical, and moral doctrines?" (133).

Background

In this era of rapid scientific advancement, human embryonic stem cell research is but one of a plethora of technologies that holds both the threat and the promise of changing the world as we know it. Embryonic stem cell research is troubling to many because of its use of human embryos, and thrilling to others for its role in the development of potentially life-saving medical therapies. Somatic cell nuclear transfer is a particularly contentious facet of stem cell research. Because it could theoretically lead to the creation of embryos sharing the exact genetic identity of an existing human being, it might lead to the custom regeneration of organs for individuals without the fear of rejection. But some fear that the existence of those genetically identical embryos might allow unscrupulous researchers to clone an existing human being should those embryos be clandestinely implanted in a willing surrogate. The potential for such manipulation of the very stuff of human life touches on fundamental questions of what it is to be human and how contemporary families and communities ought to be configured. The controversy about how, and for what purpose, to handle human embryos is concerned at its heart with determining what constitutes the beginning of human life. Although technology has made it possible for us to glimpse human life in progressively earlier stages of development, society has not yet reached agreement on the standing of the early human embryo in the face of countervailing interests. In this sense, it has been noted that the debate raging over human embryonic stem cell research mirrors "aspects of the debate over abortion rights" (Brainard 2003). Where abortion is legal, the rights of women are considered to have priority over an embryo or fetus not capable of surviving independently outside of the womb. Where human embryonic stem cell research is championed and somatic cell nuclear transfer is permitted, the rights of individuals whose lives could be made better should the promise of the research come to fruition would take precedence over the embryo, whether it is left over from fertility clinic treatments or an asexually produced blastocyst, which is the early stage embryo that is the product of somatic cell nuclear transfer.

Those who think stem cell technology would change the world for the better tout its promise to someday lead to cures for "a host of disease conditions" including "diabetes, liver and heart disease, neurodegenerative disorders such as Parkinson and Alzheimer disease, osteoporosis, blood cell disorders, muscular dystrophy, and injury caused by burns and trauma" (Lanza 2000, 1375). A very few would even welcome somatic cell nuclear transfer as a cure of last resort for infertility (Pistoi 2002, 38). Detractors warn that somatic cell nuclear transfer could too easily lead to the illegal use of embryos for reproductive purposes, (Kass 1998, 52) which virtually no society condones in light of unresolved questions of safety, efficacy, and ethics. Since somatic cell nuclear transfer involves the creation of "cloned" human embryos for the purpose of using their stem cells to regenerate diseased or damaged tissue, allowing research on the technique could introduce human embryos as a commodity into a market incapable of preventing the clandestine implantation of cloned embryos for reproductive purposes. Even if their use were successfully restricted to research, the destruction of embryos for their stem cells (derived during the blastocyst stage, when embryos consist of between 64 and 200 cells (Nuland 2002)) would still be an anathema to many. Critics who fear that stem cell research and other biotechnologies will bring about a "posthuman future" where social relations and human nature are fundamentally altered (Wade 2002a) seem hopelessly at odds with advocates of scientific freedom and those seeking cures for a multitude of debilitating diseases. So, to the many intractable moral, ethical, and scientific challenges posed by human embryonic stem cell research can be added the political challenge it presents as citizens with divergent views struggle to gain priority in the policy-making process.

Methodology

This analysis will apply two facets of John Rawls' construct of political liberalism to a consideration of the human embryonic stem cell research controversy. Since the philosophical construct of political liberalism is intricate and extensive and the space for this analysis is limited, it will focus on two pertinent aspects of political liberalism. The first is drawn from the first stage of Rawls' "exposition of justice as fairness"—the cornerstone of political liberalism—"as a freestanding view addressed to" the question just posed: "how is it possible that there can be a stable and just society whose free and equal citizens are deeply divided by conflicting and even incommensurable religious, philosophical and moral doctrines?" The first stage details the answer to this question by describing the "basic structure" of such a society as one regulated by a shared political conception of justice serving as "the basis of public reason in debates about political questions when constitutional essentials and matters of basic justice are at stake" (48). While ideas of the reasonable and the rational are fundamental to this basic structure, certain limits to public reason—described as "burdens of judgment"—are acknowledged. These burdens of judgment outline key "sources, or causes, of disagreement between reasonable persons" (55). A utopian conception, political liberalism depends upon actors who are not only rational, but who are, perhaps more importantly, reasonable. Reasonable people are defined as those who "take into account the consequences of their actions on others' well-being" and "can cooperate with others on terms all can accept" (49f and 50). The fact that political liberalism admits of six significant and weighty "burdens of judgment" even with rational, reasonable actors as a given can seem cause for skepticism that such a society can exist. The case of human embryonic stem cell research and the attendant question of cloning offer an illustration of just how burdensome those burdens of judgment can be.

The second facet of political liberalism employed in this analysis is drawn from the "second stage of the exposition," which "considers how the well-ordered democratic society of justice as fairness may establish and preserve unity and stability given the reasonable pluralism characteristic of it" (134). The concept of "overlapping consensus of reasonable comprehensive doctrines" provides assurance that even in the face of controversial and divisive issues such as stem cell research, "a well-ordered society can be unified and stable" (134). A reasonable comprehensive doctrine is defined as "an exercise of theoretical reason … covering the major religious, philosophical and moral aspects of human life," which employs both theoretical and practical reason in balancing conflicting values, and "normally belongs to, or draws upon, a tradition of thought or doctrine" (59). Where it is possible for such doctrines to overlap, though they may endorse many disparate conceptions of the good, is upon their shared political conception, endorsed by "each from its own point of view" (134). The case of stem cell research, characterized by conflicting comprehensive doctrines, may ultimately be resolved in the realm of this "most reasonable basis of social unity" and "basic idea of political liberalism" (134): overlapping consensus.

Discussion

In order to understand the concept of overlapping consensus as it applies to the controversy over stem cell research, it is essential to first outline who holds the reasonable comprehensive doctrines expected to overlap in order for consensus to be achieved in accordance with the model of political liberalism. These doctrines, though strictly delineated, nevertheless allow for consensus because, according to Rawls' model, they are reasonable and find agreement on a political conception of justice. Although beset by onerous burdens of judgments, overlapping consensus of reasonable comprehensive doctrines is seen as possible within the framework of political liberalism.

Comprehensive Doctrines

With political liberalism as a framework, stakeholders in the human embryonic stem cell research policy process can best be described as those individuals who subscribe to the different comprehensive doctrines that espouse the various views and values fueling the debate. A fully comprehensive doctrine "includes conceptions of what is of value in human life, and ideals of personal character, as well as ideals of friendship and of familial and associational relationships, and much else that is to inform our conduct" (13). Even when a doctrine is only partially comprehensive, comprising "a number of, but by no means all, nonpolitical values and virtues and is rather loosely articulated," it is taken to play the same role in the framework as a fully comprehensive doctrine in shaping the mind set of its adherents.

Religious groups are perhaps the easiest to see in terms of subscribing to comprehensive doctrines, and of course several religious groups figure prominently in the stem cell research and cloning debate. The Roman Catholic Church, whose doctrine advocates the respect "of human life in all its stages" (Fitzgerald 2002) and currently teaches that life begins at the moment of conception and ends with natural death, seeks a ban on all such research for either reproductive or therapeutic purposes. On this issue, the Catholic Church is in accord with conservative Protestant denominations—including evangelicals and fundamentalists—who believe that "the creation and destruction of human embryos for research purposes is immoral" (Taylor 2002). Jewish theologians, on the other hand, can be said to support embryonic stem cell research, including somatic cell nuclear transfer or "therapeutic cloning," citing their potential to relieve or heal suffering from disease—"a strong imperative in Jewish tradition." (Taylor 2002). Also, "unlike most Christian denominations, Jews" give status neither "to a fetus during its first 40 days of gestation" nor to "an embryo outside of a woman." (Taylor 2002). In 2001, the year in which President Bush wrote an Executive Order banning the use of federal funds for the research, "the nation's largest Orthodox Jewish organizations declared their support ... for allowing scientists to clone human embryos for medical research, breaking with conservative Christian groups" on the topic (Cooperman 2002).

Philosophical and moral doctrines are also defined as comprehensive doctrines, though they are more likely to be partially comprehensive and somewhat more difficult to conceptualize or categorize. Figuring prominently in the stem cell policy arena are proponents of science and research whose worldview seems significantly shaped by the conviction that scientific means most often lead to morally justifiable ends. Those sharing this philosophy support virtually all stem cell research, including somatic cell nuclear transfer, and some might be willing to consider the prospect of pursuing reproductive cloning should the science someday give reason for encouragement in this regard. (Nevertheless, it is believed that techniques employed to successfully clone "mice, sheep and other animals ... would 'have to be modified' to make it work on primates, including humans" (Pearson 2003).

Doctors' and researchers' groups, such as the American Medical Association, the Federation of American Societies for Experimental Biology, the American College of Obstetricians and Gynecologists, and patient advocacy groups, such as the Coalition for the Advancement of Medical Research, the Juvenile Diabetes Research Foundation, and the Parkinson's Action Network, are but a few of those more traditionally defined as interest groups who could nonetheless be said to embrace a pro-science comprehensive doctrine.

Environmentalists could also be said to share a philosophy arguably definable as a partially comprehensive doctrine. Their doctrine advocates protection and preservation of the earth, respect for all living things, and balance in nature. Where biotechnology is concerned, they oppose everything from "genetically modified crops (known derisively as 'Frankenfoods')" to "genetic enhancement (inserting supposedly desirable genes into embryos)" and human cloning of any type (Henig 2003). Environmental groups such as the Friends of the Earth, the Sierra Club, and Greenpeace, U.S.A. oppose "not research on cloned embryos but what may come next: the genetic modification and enhancement of humans" (Weiss 2002).

These are just a few of the reasonable comprehensive doctrines whose views and value judgments play a role in the stem cell policy-making process. "A society may also contain unreasonable and irrational, and even mad, comprehensive doctrines. In their case the problem is to contain them so that they do not undermine the unity and justice of society" (Rawls 1993, xviii). The Raelians, a "sect that believes space travelers created the human race by cloning" and made unsubstantiated claims in 2002 "that it had produced the first human clone," (Canedy 2002) may be the field's most likely candidate for a crazy, though so far relatively harmless, doctrine. As for the abundance of reasonable comprehensive doctrines, the fact that they are so disparate and seemingly irreconcilable is not perceived by political liberalism as a "disaster but rather as the natural outcome of activities of human reason under enduring free institutions" (Rawls 1993, xxvi).

Reason and its Limits: The Burdens of Judgment

Political liberalism expects that "a modern democratic society" will be characterized by a pluralism of comprehensive doctrines, which, though incompatible, can coexist because they are reasonable (Rawls 1993, xxvi). "The ideal of public reason," so central to political liberalism, "does not often lead to general agreement of views, nor should it" (lvii). Indeed, Rawls says that the expectation that "social unity and concord requires agreement" on some particular doctrine is a hallmark of "intolerance," the weakening of which "helps to clear the way for liberal institutions" (xxvii). It is expected that reasonable people, defined above as those who "take into account the consequences of their actions on others' well-being" and who "can cooperate with others on terms all can accept," (49f and 50) will employ public reasoning when "some political decision must be made, as with legislators enacting laws and judges deciding cases" (liv). In such circumstances, "all must be able to reasonably endorse the process by which" that political decision is made (lv).

There are, of course, limits to the reconciliation that can be achieved by public reason. Rawls describes these limits as deriving from several broad categories, including "those resulting from citizens' conflicting comprehensive doctrines … and those resulting from the burdens of judgment" (lx). This analysis will focus on the burdens of judgment—which are encountered even when those judging are fully reasonable. The stem cell policy-making process and forum for public consensus are rife with such burdens.

The first burden of judgment occurs when "the evidence—empirical and scientific—bearing on the case is conflicting and complex, and thus hard to assess and evaluate" (56). The science of stem cell research, and somatic cell nuclear transfer, in particular, is clearly complex. Whether for reproductive or therapeutic purposes, the process of

177

somatic cell nuclear transfer begins by "taking the nucleus from a patient's cell and implanting it into a human egg cell that (has) had its nucleus removed" (Lanza). The resulting egg cell with its new nucleus is then stimulated "to divide to produce a blastocyst embryo" (Weissman). For therapeutic purposes, the cells from this embryo are then coaxed "to produce stem cell lines ... Such stem cells are unspecialized cells that can develop into almost all kinds of body cells" to "regenerate damaged tissues" (Weissman). For reproductive purposes, the resulting blastocyst would be "placed into a uterus" and allowed to continue developing "with the intent of creating a newborn" (Weissman). Neither therapeutic nor reproductive cloning has yet been achieved in humans. "Despite optimistic statements about curing diseases, almost all researchers, when questioned, confess that such accomplishments are more dream than reality" (Kolata 2003). Because stem cell research is still a nascent technology, scientists themselves are in the process of assessing and evaluating the science. Policy makers and the public most often must struggle to make sense of it all.

The second burden of judgment states that, "even where we are fully in agreement about the kinds of considerations that are relevant, we may disagree about their weight, and so arrive at different judgments" (Rawls 1993, 56). Although most agree that the status of the human embryo is the pivotal consideration where embryonic stem cell research is concerned, various reasonable actors are of differing opinions as to the nature of that status and the weight it should be accorded. Should the potential of the human embryo to develop into human life preclude its use for research purposes? Or would it be wrong not to pursue the "promising new lines of inquiry made possible by embryonic stem cells?" (Wade 2002b).

Third, according to Rawls, to the "extent all our concepts ... are vague and subject to hard cases ... this indeterminacy means that we must rely on judgment and interpretation ... within some range ... where reasonable persons may differ" (56). Definitional distinctions resulting from varying interpretations that come into play in the stem cell research debate create a particularly vexing burden of judgment. Although the term "therapeutic cloning," once favored by stem cell researchers, highlights the potentially curative properties of the procedure, "human embryonic cloning," favored by abortion opponents, underscores its origins (Wade 2002c). "Nuclear transplantation (or transferal) to produce human pluripotent stem cell lines," a phrase favored by Stanford researchers, takes the cloning terminology off the table all together, whereas the product of this procedure is emphatically denoted a "cloned human embryo" by the President's Council on Bioethics (Wade 2002c). To some, the product of nuclear transfer is none other than a cloned human embryo; to others, this product of a form of parthenogenesis is a replication of something other than a new life form altogether. The vast array of conflicting value-laden terminology exacerbates the challenges posed by the complexity of the science and the weighing of relevant moral and ethical considerations, making identification, interpretation, and judgment of the facts difficult, and divergent judgments by reasonable people more likely.

The fourth burden of judgment is essentially a restatement of the adage "where you stand depends upon where you sit." Given citizens' different life experiences, ethnicities, social groups, and work experience, it is natural, as Rawls says, "for their judgments to diverge, at least to some degree, on many if not most cases of any significant complexity" (57). This source of diverging judgments is distinct from conflicting comprehensive doctrines, which are in a category by themselves. Although they also result in divergent judgments, conflicting comprehensive doctrines have the values held by citizens at their heart, while this particular burden of judgment results from their different stations in life. For instance, where stem cell research is concerned, the poor may be less inclined to seek, or be able to afford, medical therapies derived from the research should any such therapies eventually be realized. Their necessarily more immediate concern with the availability of affordable health care *now* will color their interest in or support for research on hypothetical stem cell therapies in the face of a very real and pressing need. Social justice is just one of the many ethical concerns raised by stem cell research (McLean 2002). It is also just one of the many considerations raised by the fourth burden of judgment.

The fact that "there are different kinds of normative considerations of different force on both sides of an issue," making it difficult to form "an overall assessment," constitutes the fifth burden of judgment (McLean 2002). Conservatives defending the virtue and normality of the nuclear family fear that reproductive cloning made possible by somatic cell nuclear transfer could become just another venue for the dismantling of traditional family structures, and so oppose stem cell research of any kind. If the dreaded slippery slope should ever lead to the reality of reproductive cloning, they "favor limiting cloning to intact, heterosexual families." (Wilson 1998, 99). On the other side of the issue, homosexuals wishing to become parents might find somatic cell nuclear transfer an appealing way to parent a child to whom they exclusively have genetic ties and would thus favor the advancement of such research. It is hard to imagine any reconciliation of normative views between these two opposite camps.

Finally, Rawls notes "any system of social institutions is limited in the values it can admit so that some selection made from the full range of moral and political values might be realized" (57). This sixth burden of judgment points out that we are "forced to select among cherished values, or when we hold several ... we must restrict each in view of the requirements of others" (57). This sometimes results in bargains that leave participants feeling compromised. If discontent is deep enough, the issue is likely to percolate up through the political process again until a more satisfactory compromise is achieved. President Bush's August 2001 decision to allow federally funded research on existing stem cell lines, but banning the use of federal funds to establish new lines, created discontent on both sides of the issue. Those finding the use of human embryos for research unpalatable could still be offended, and researchers found themselves bridling at restrictions on their scientific work. Since the moral status of human embryos remains unresolved and recent scientific developments provide further evidence that the inability to "use the newly derived, latest and best cell lines ... puts us at a disadvantage," (Weiss 2003) it was only a matter of time before the administration's policy was reexamined. President Obama's decision in early 2009 to rescind President Bush's Executive Order now allows the use of federal funds for research on existing stem cell lines. Nonetheless, it does not allow the creation of "patient-specific" stem cells sought through research using somatic cell nuclear transfer, which is restricted by the Dickey-Wicker amendment banning any destruction of human embryos.

Although it is easy to find in the burdens of judgment cause for despair that the policy process will ever reach resolution, Rawls actually defines "the willingness to recognize the burdens of judgment and to accept their consequences for the use of public reason in directing the legitimate exercise of political power in a constitutional regime" as one of the two "basic aspects of the reasonable" (54). The other is "the willingness to propose fair terms of cooperation and to abide by them provided others do." Thus, rather than acting as an impediment to the principles of justice, the burdens of judgment are integral to their basic structure.

Overlapping Consensus

The first stage of the exposition put forth by Rawls in Political Liberalism lays down the structure of a society in which public reason prevails, in response to the question, "how is it possible for there to exist over time a just and stable society of free and equal citizens, who remain profoundly divided by reasonable religious, philosophical and moral doctrines?" The second stage describes the mechanisms that make it possible. In a word—or two—it is achieved by overlapping consensus. This overlapping consensus of the reasonable comprehensive doctrines held by citizens occurs in the realm of the political, not on the more limited terrain of one or another comprehensive doctrine alone.

The concept of overlapping consensus rests upon the presumption of reasonable pluralism. It is expected that reasonable, rational individuals in a society will naturally embrace different doctrines and reach different conclusions on matters of importance. But these same reasonable, rational citizens are also understood to share a political conception of justice in which no one comprehensive doctrine can be preeminent. So Roman Catholics, Protestants, and Jews, and environmentalists, scientists, and their supporters endorse the power of the government and its laws as a collective body of free and equal citizens living according to the liberal principle of legitimacy, whereby they endorse the use of political power exercised in accordance with a constitution agreed upon by all.

If we are to accept that political questions can be resolved "by appeal to political values alone" rather than reliance on the dictums of diverse comprehensive doctrines, then political values must have "sufficient weight to override all other values that may come in conflict with them" (Rawls 1993, 138). Given the sampling of comprehensive doctrines above and the myriad deeply held values intrinsic to them, this seems almost too much to ask. Yet Rawls offers reassurance that "political values are very great values and hence not easily overridden"; in the words of John Stuart Mill, they provide "the very groundwork of our existence" (139). The virtues of political cooperation make a constitutional regime possible and constitute part of society's political capital by underpinning an array of values of justice including "the values of equal political and civil liberty; fair equality of opportunity; the values of economic reciprocity; the social bases of mutual respect between citizens" and the values of pubic reason (Rawls 1993, 139).

Rawls' construct of political liberalism describes citizens as "moral agents" with a "capacity for a conception of justice and a capacity for a conception of the good" (19). The moral sensibility that imbues the reasonable comprehensive doctrines embraced by citizens also infuses their political conception. Although some moral doctrines contain an element not admitting of compromise, political liberalism "does not aim to replace comprehensive doctrines, religious or nonreligious, but intends to be equally distinct from both and, it hopes, acceptable to both" (Rawls 1993, xl). The overlapping consensus of reasonable doctrines necessary for political liberalism to thrive finds a fit between the political conception, in itself a moral conception, and the comprehensive views of the citizens sharing that political conception. Public recognition of the great values of the political virtues informs that vital consensus.

Although the burdens of judgment as illustrated by the human embryonic stem cell controversy seem cause for concern that reconciliation among reasonable views might ever be achieved, their very existence also underscores the need for political liberalism, which "takes to heart the absolute depth of that irreconcilable latent conflict" (Rawls 1993, xxviii). Without it, how could such radically distinct views peaceably coexist? A shared political conception informed by public reason and achieved by an overlapping consensus of reasonable comprehensive doctrines ultimately makes it possible for a just and free society to exist "under conditions of deep doctrinal conflict with no prospect of resolution" (Rawls 1993, xxx).

Policy Recommendations

An examination of the human embryonic stem cell research controversy through the lens of political liberalism suggests three courses of action to assist in mitigating the potential of such controversies to create social unrest. The first, brought to mind by the model of political liberalism, is to initiate measures to strengthen civic education. Only if the virtues and values of the shared political conception of constitutional democracy are reiterated and renewed by each generation can it hope to endure. The second, suggested by the scientific complexity of stem cell and other modern technologies, is to promote the virtues of science education and ensure that it keeps pace with scientific advancement. A public incapable of understanding the dramatic and at times morally confounding advances of modern science will find it challenging to reach consensus of any kind on issues about which it is ill informed. The third is to carefully consider the international implications of making stem cell policy. Although Rawls' construct of political liberalism assumes a closed model—taken to mean an individual nation or society—we are all, it has frequently been noted of late, citizens of the world—part of a global community. International boundaries are increasingly incapable of containing scientific technologies; those banned in one nation may be easily accessible to its citizens in another. The benefits realized or ill effects inflicted on society by stem cell technology or any other scientific advancement will ultimately not be limited to the residents of isolated countries. A new model of political philosophy will be needed to conceptualize how consensus might be achieved on an international level to use the promise of scientific advancement to the best advantage of all people.

Conclusion

When particularly divisive, intractable topics appear on the political agenda, it is natural for some hand wringing to occur over whether consensus might ever be achieved. At such times it is useful to reflect on theories of political philosophy that may offer reassurance of the resilience of our constitutional democracy, provide a framework for more in-depth analysis of the issue at hand, and perhaps even suggest relevant policy recommendations. Although political liberalism as outlined by Rawls is a utopian conception based on an elegant model at times somewhat removed from reality, it nonetheless provides a framework for classifying and explicating sources of controversy—the burdens of judgment—and outlines a road map towards reconciliation achieved by overlapping consensus.

References

Brainard, Jeffrey. 2003. "House votes to ban research cloning—Again," *Chronicle of Higher Education*, February 28, available at website for the Coalition for the Advancement of Medical Research (CAMR) http://www.camradvocacy.org/fastaction/news.asp?id=522.

Canedy, Dana and Kenneth Chang. 2002. "Sect Claims First Cloned Baby," *The New York Times*, 28 December.

Cooperman, Alan. 2002. "2 Jewish Groups Back Therapeutic Cloning," *The Washington Post*, 13 March 2002, sec. A4.

Fitzgerald, Father Kevin T. 2002. Testimony before the United States Senate Committee on the Judiciary, *Human Cloning: Must We Sacrifice Medical Research in the Name of a Total Ban?* 5 February.

Henig, Robin Marantz. 2003. "Deciding When Science Has Gone Astray," *The New York Times*, 25 February, available fromhttp://www.nytimes.com/2003/02/25/science/25REGU.html?pagewanted=1.

Kass, Leon R. 1998. "The Wisdom of Repugnance," In *The Ethics of Human Cloning*. Washington, DC: The AEI Press.

Kolata, Gina. 2003. "The Promise of Therapeutic Cloning," *The New York Times*, 5 January.

Lanza, Robert B., Arthur L. Kaplan, Lee M. Silver, Jose B. Cibelli, Michael D. West, and Ronald M. Green. 2000. "The Ethical Validity of Using Nuclear Transfer in Human Transplantation," *The Journal of the American Medical Association*, 284 (2000): 1375.

McLean, Margaret R. 2002. "'What's in a Name?' Nuclear Transplantation and the Ethics of Stem Cell Research," *Hastings Law Journal* 53 (July).

Nuland, Sherwin B. 2002. "Send In No Clones," *The New York Times*, 17 November.

Pearson, Helen. 2003. "Human clones doomed?" *Nature*, 11 April, available from http://www.nature.com/news/2003/030407/full/news030407-12.html.

Pistoi, Sergio. "Father of impossible children: Ignoring nearly universal opprobrium, Sevorino Antinori presses ahead with plans to clone a human being," *Scientific American* 286 (April 2002): 38.

John Rawls. 1993. *Political Liberalism*. New York: Columbia University Press.

Taylor, Leah. 2002. "Seeing double: the cloning conundrum," *Canadian Speeches* 16 (November—December).

Wade, Nicholas. 2002a. "A Dim View of a 'Posthuman Future'" *The New York Times*, 2 April, sec. D1.

Wade, Nicholas. 2002b. "New Stanford Institute is to Study Controversial Stem Cell Manipulation," *The New York Times*, 12 December.

Wade, Nicholas. 2002c. "Word war breaks out in research on stem cells," *The New York Times*, 21 December.

Weiss, Rick. 2002. "Cloning creates odd bedfellows," *The Washington Post*, February 10, sec. B1.

Weiss, Rick. 2003. "Stem Cell Strides Test Bush Policy; Scientists Push for Use of Newer Cell Colonies," *The Washington Post*, 22 April, sec. A1.

Wilson, James O. 1998. "Sex and Family," In *The Ethics of Human Cloning* Washington, DC: The AEI Press.

Weissman, Irving. 2002. Testimony before the United States Senate Committee on the Judiciary, *Human Cloning: Must We Sacrifice Medical Research in the Name of a Total Ban?* 25 February.

New Patterns of Political Patronage and their Effect on Health Policy

Susan J. Tolchin, *George Mason University*
Debasree Das Gupta, *George Mason University*
Jeffrey Beck, *George Mason University*

Introduction

New York's billionaire mayor, Michael Bloomberg, once mentioned "[S]ome people, when they want something from somebody, walk up and hit them with a two by four, I walk up and give them hugs and kisses." That is the way the world works— usually—in politics and government, in business communities, and even in families. There are many definitions of politics, including "the art of the possible" and "the art of compromise." But as Jake Arvey, the late Illinois Democratic leader who fostered Adlai Stevenson's political career, said, "Politics is the art of putting people under obligation to you."[1] Politicians put people under obligation to them through patronage, which cements loyalty up and down the political ladder; patronage is the awarding of discretionary favors in government in exchange for political support. Most important, it can also deprive recipients of their ability to make independent decisions.

Patronage affects policy at all levels of government: cities, states, and at the federal level. It is beginning even to drive U.S. foreign policy, often in ways that potentially undermine America's stature in the world.[2] Patronage is a neutral concept that can be used in positive as well as negative ways. Indeed, nowhere is this ambivalence more evident than in the case of health and healthcare policy. Many politicians have blocked the construction of health facilities and hospitals in deserving neighborhoods to punish opponents.

At other times, patronage connections have been used to successfully earmark millions of dollars for health research in the interest of finding cures for specific diseases. Most recently, patronage has been given a new opportunity to expand, primarily through the new hybrid organizations being created through the Obama administration's effort at healthcare reform. Such organizations (including health option exchanges and new oversight organizations) represent perfect opportunities for a further expansion of patronage into the healthcare system in the United States.

Over the years, elected officials and government organizations have engaged in countless patronage practices, thereby violating the basic expectation of the American electorate.[3] Health politics stands out for the new opportunities presented by changes in the law. What follows are examples of how current examples of political patronage

---

[1] All direct quotes in this article that are not cited as notes are drawn from interviews. More than 200 people were interviewed in researching patronage practices in U.S. politics. The article is excerpted from Tolchin, Martin and Susan J. Tolchin, *Pinstripe Patronage: Political Favoritism from the Clubhouse to the White House and Beyond* (Boulder, CO: Paradigm Publishers, 2011).

[2] Private corporations that represent the United States in Iraq and Afghanistan have committed abuses that have outraged the local citizenry, and undermined the nation's ability to act in ways that are vital to its interests.

[3] See Tolchin and Tolchin (2011) for a detailed review.

encourage public officials to compromise the public's interests for private and/or political gain. Patronage practices often operate with more subtlety than cases of outright corruption, when the legal system steps in to halt the abuses.

The Range of Patronage Politics

New York's Mayor Bloomberg successfully used his patronage connections to overcome opposition from the owners of restaurants and bars and persuade the city council to outlaw smoking in public spaces. Without this support as well as his political connections, it would have been far more difficult for the mayor to get the smoking ban passed. Another prominent example of patronage involved a former Michigan Governor Jim Blanchard, who had been appointed Ambassador to Canada by President Clinton. Blanchard was not surprised when his phone rang at the start of the 2008 presidential primary season, and a raspy voice intoned "Mr. Ambassador, we need your help." How could he refuse Bill Clinton? Blanchard explained that "I've had a 20 year relationship with the Clintons," adding, "I'm intensely loyal." Blanchard became a strong advocate for Hillary Clinton's campaign for the Democratic nomination for President and even represented her before the Democratic Party's Rules Committee. Many such personal favors accrued to Clinton as a result of his patronage connections. Yet, he was unable to shore up enough Congressional support to pass his health reform legislation. Indeed, savvy political leaders like Clinton often have to learn the hard way about the limitations of patronage when it comes to advancing policy goals. President Obama was more successful than President Clinton at getting a new healthcare reform law. Rather than use standard patronage practices to get the law passed, the Obama administration gave Congress "guidance" and managed to get the law passed by "encouraging" the party to influence Representatives and Senators to vote for the law. This new law, however, presents new opportunities for patronage. Several examples include a new layer of bureaucracy in the federal government to manage the law and the potential creation of hybrid organizations.

In the United States, political favors come in many forms—from a mayor's attendance at a wedding, to a governor's speech at a private dinner, to a President's invitation to spend a night in the Lincoln bedroom. More substantial favors include zoning variances, tax exemptions, judgeships, refereeships, appointments to boards and commissions, guardianships, insurance contracts, and bank deposits. The successful patronage seeker is well aware that the government must bank its money, insure its property, and construct office buildings—all on a noncompetitive basis because bank and insurance rates are uniform and there are no objective standards for architecture, engineering, and (often) construction contracts. Those who were "selected" can expect to be called upon for future campaign contributions, and were probably selected in the first place for their past generosity. Most important, city and state controllers reap political power by deciding where to invest government funds. Government buildings need furniture, stationery, plumbing systems, heating, wiring, and vending machines— franchises often worth millions of dollars to the recipients of this patronage. In the implementation of the new health insurance law, many opportunities for patronage exist—especially and until the various facets of the law become known and blanketed into the civil service system.

186

At times, a politician will block a patronage request to settle a score or deny a neighborhood project to punish opponents. Such patronage practices affect the quality of life of most Americans and negatively impact community health and home values. Former Mayor Adrian Fenty of Washington, DC, openly rewarded his supporters in the City Council with projects in their districts, while withholding funds from districts represented by political opponents. After his reelection in 1973, Mayor John Lindsay of New York jokingly denied being a practitioner of this strategy. At the 1974 dinner of the Inner Circle, a group of political reporters, he said, "[H]ow can Queens (a county that voted for his opponent) complain that I haven't given them any new facilities? My new budget clearly shows plans to build a sewage treatment plant there." Of course, a sewage treatment plant is not exactly the kind of public works project sought by most neighborhoods! (Tolchin and Tolchin 1972, 29).

Old-fashioned patronage practices have changed very little. In addition, politicians today have opportunities undreamed of by George Washington Plunkitt, the colorful turn-of-the-century Tammany boss, and his political heirs.[4] Today's Plunkitts can choose among a vast array of favors for loyalists. Through privatization, a public official is freed from the judicial constraints on his ability to reward supporters with government jobs and noncompetitive contracts. A mayor can pick up the telephone and find a job for a supporter in a hospital or engineering company that has benefited from his largesse. The tools of patronage have changed since the glory days of the old political machines, whose leaders happily dispensed food for the poor and jobs for ward heelers.

In addition to traditional patronage, the new landscape now includes "pinstripe patronage"—billions of dollars in outsourcing many functions that were previously conducted by government. Healthcare is one of the many functions not envisaged by the Founding Fathers, and therefore a leading candidate for outsourcing. Pinstripe patronage also includes earmarks, tucked into legislation by influential members of Congress, as well as appointments to executive positions or places on the boards of the numerous hybrid agencies like Fannie Mae and Freddie Mac that now dot the political landscape. Pinstripe patronage usually benefits those more at home in a boardroom than on an assembly line, who then reciprocate by giving politicians the ever-increasing funds needed to conduct political campaigns. Pinstripe patronage has replaced the Christmas turkey and snow removal jobs that politicians gave the less fortunate, and includes billions of dollars in noncompetitive contracts.[5] State and local governments followed suit, with soaring budgets for both privatization and "earmarks" that all too often rewarded political supporters. Defense department contracts dwarf those awarded by state and local government.

---

[4] Plunkitt represented the 15th Senate District of New York City. See William L. Riordan, *Plunkitt of Tammany Hall*, originally published in 1905 (New York: Bedford Books of St. Martin's Press, 1994 edition).

[5] Such no-bid contracts have been awarded to private companies like Halliburton and Blackwater whose executives have given substantial contributions to both political parties. Today, it is estimated that more than 50 percent of all federal functions are "contracted out," most of them without competitive bidding. In the fiscal year 2006, the U.S. government spent more than $415 billion on contracts with 176,172 companies. About one-quarter of that total, $100 billion, went to only six companies. More than 60 percent of these contracts, most of them with the Department of Defense, were awarded without competitive bidding. "The rapid growth in no-bid and limited competition contracts has made full and open competition the exception, not the rule," reported Robert O'Harrow. See Robert O'Harrow, "Federal No-Bid Contracts on Rise," *Washington Post*, August 22, 2007, 1.

The enormous growth of government in the last century created a concurrent expansion of the discretionary powers of political leaders.[6] Welcomed equally by Democrats and Republicans, the new patronage opportunities increased their ability to reward constituents and remained the lifeblood of politics and government. Patronage exists at all levels of government, including school boards, healthcare organizations, county commissions, city and state administrations, Congress, the judiciary, and the White House. A President's vast patronage powers explain why he almost always controls his party. Barring an overriding national issue, patronage powers, usually vested in party elders, explain why politics is usually oriented more to the past than to current movements, and more toward conservative than to innovative programs. Congress especially rewards longevity with power, allowing those with long service to collect numerous IOUs and to obtain the lion's share of new ones. Even those members motivated by ideological commitment quickly discover, in the words of the legendary Speaker of the House, Sam Rayburn of Texas, "[T]o get along, you have to go along" (Tolchin and Tolchin 1972, 187).

Patronage powers also give politicians the power to determine the quality of law enforcement, one of the most coveted powers of government. The discretionary aspects of law enforcement often surface when a new administration prosecutes public officials who previously enjoyed immunity while their own party controlled the administration. Few Presidents have used these powers in a more partisan manner than George W. Bush, whose attorney general fired prosecutors considered overly aggressive in pursuing Republican officials and too sluggish in prosecuting Democrats (Eggen and Kane 2007; Johnson 2008).

Earmarks and Other Patronage Practices

Old-fashioned patronage practices—such as placing supporters in non-exempt government jobs—continued to thrive well into the twenty-first century. Indeed, examples of political patronage can be found in every state. Although some of its practitioners have recently wound up behind bars, many experts believe that the system is deeply embedded in the culture of many communities. "The Jacksonian ideal was that patronage was efficient," said Prof. Alvin S. Felzenberg of the University of Pennsylvania. "It ensured accountability because public dissatisfaction with the delivery of services inevitably led to a politician's vulnerability at the polls." Movers and shakers in politics have long used patronage to achieve their goals. President Franklin Delano Roosevelt, for example, created a raft of alphabet agencies, which became patronage havens. Instead, he could have placed these agencies in existing cabinet departments whose employees were subject to civil service laws (Tolchin and Tolchin 1972, 257-258).

In more recent times politicians continue to reward supporters even when five decisions by the U.S. Supreme Court placed severe restrictions on hiring, firing, and promoting government employees, as well as awarding government contracts, on the

---

[6] Today, the federal workforce comprises of 1.9 million permanent full-time civil servants: a size that is about the same as it was in 1960. Yet, an additional 7.6 million contract employees have been added to the federal payroll, according to Max Stier, President and CEO of the nonpartisan Partnership for Public Services. While the federal government, albeit purportedly, was reducing its workforce through privatization and contracting out, employment in state and local government—about 80,000 entities including states, counties, special water districts, and sewer districts—almost tripled during the same period.

basis of party affiliation and political support.[7] The Court ignored warnings from many quarters that patronage was the lifeblood of politics and government. Many assumed that these decisions would have sounded the death knell of political patronage. Not so. Nature abhors a vacuum, and despite all the new laws against "politics as usual," the empty spaces were quickly filled. In other words, patronage did not go away; it just took new forms. Today, patronage lives on, often in disguise, thanks to soaring government budgets and the phenomenal increase of earmarks on the local, state, and federal level for everything from the arts and sciences to the infamous "Bridge to Nowhere."[8] At the same time, there has been a great increase in privatization, outsourcing everything from state hospitals, prisons, and transportation to the war in Iraq.[9] These efforts have been expanded further on both the state and national level through recent efforts in several states and nationwide at healthcare reform. Such efforts often include new positions within the state and national governments as well as abundant opportunities for new contracts and new hybrid organizations to help implement the new policies. As a result, earmarks, privatization, and reform have provided grist for the patronage mill.

According to some estimates, earmarks constitute less than 1–2 percent of the federal budget. Even 1 percent of the federal budget is not a small number and amounts to about $38 billion. Legislators often use earmarks to reward their constituents. During his tenure in Congress, Rahm Emanuel (2007) (D-Illinois) secured earmarks to support a children's hospital facility, fund after-school and teacher training programs, rebuild bridges and provide computers for police patrol cars. In 2009, earmarks were front and center of the mammoth bailout bill. Although Democratic senators supported this $700 billion bill, some of them were nonetheless aided by "incentives." Republican Senator Arlen Specter, who switched his allegiance to the Democratic Party, provided the 60th vote that was needed to avoid a filibuster. In return he negotiated a $10 billion increase in the National Institute of Health budget for biomedical research as the price of his vote.

Oftentimes, earmarks provide society with a rewarding outcome. Years before the isolation of the Cystic Fibrosis (CF) gene, the Government Affairs Committee of the Cystic Fibrosis Foundation lobbied Congress for an earmark for CF research. In 1988, the same year in which the CF gene was discovered, Representative Silvio Conte (R-Massachusetts) introduced in the appropriations bill an earmark of $6 million for CF research.[10] Today, appropriations for CF research are in excess of $80 million, funds that further research in the effort to find a cure for CF.

In some instances, patronage practices amounted to clear cases of corruption. The legendary governor Huey Long of Louisiana would often boast openly, "I steal money, but a lot of what I stole has spilled over in no-toll bridges, hospitals and to build [a] university [Louisiana State University]." Another example involves the University of

---

[7] The five U.S. Supreme Court decisions were: *Elrod v. Burns* (1976), 509 F. 2d 1133, *Branti v. Finkel* (1980), 445 U.S. 507, *Rutan v. Republican Party of Illinois* (1990), 42 U.S. 62, *Board of County Commissioners, Wabaunsee County, Kansas v. Umbehr* (1996), 518 US 668, and *O'Hare Truck Service v. City of Northlake* (1996), Ill. 518 US 712.

[8] In 2005, the late Senator Ted Stevens of Alaska had sponsored Alaska's infamous $433 million "Bridge to Nowhere" earmark. The project proposed to build two bridges that would have connected two remote islands to the Alaskan mainland. The "Bridge to Nowhere" was eventually abandoned, thanks to the public outcry over what was regarded as a frivolous use of taxpayer dollars.

[9] Although privatization, outsourcing, and contracting out are somewhat different conceptually, they are used interchangeably in this essay because there is considerable overlap from the patronage point of view.

[10] Full disclosure: co-author Susan Tolchin testified on behalf of obtaining those funds.

Medicine and Dentistry of New Jersey (UMDNJ). In fact, the University almost lost its accreditation when it was revealed that many of its administrators and physicians were appointed on the basis of their political connections, and not their competence. The University was responsible for scores of job opportunities to New Jersey politicians. "The University of Medicine and Dentistry is a microcosm of corruption in the rest of the Garden State. It created a system that assigned numbers to job applicants based on their political connections" (Margolin and Heyboer 2005).[11] What was even more shocking was that students were admitted on the basis of their patronage relationships, and that politicians would all too often pressurize the University to give passing grades to those medical students who had failed their standardized tests. The UMDNJ also became the center of an investigation for Medicare fraud in 2005. The University's Board of Directors was given a choice by the U.S. attorney, then Chris Christie, to either be taken over by a federal guardian or face a federal indictment of $4.9 million. The University chose the former option.

Patronage in Public and Hybrid Agencies

The economic debacle of 2008–2010 brought government back as a major player. But before the crisis struck, government as we know it had changed. Today, government on all levels has become so "lean" that contractors are often used to fill the void. In fact, contractors and "hybrid" or quasi-governmental agencies far exceed what we used to think of as government; their functions range far beyond what the Founding Fathers envisaged, even considering how different life is today from what it was in 1789. Indeed, contracting has virtually become a "fourth branch of the government." The current federal workforce is the same as it was in 1960 and stands at 1.9 million permanent, full-time civil servants. But what most Americans do not know is that their tax dollars were spent to pay an additional 7.6 million contract employees who were also on the federal payroll.[12] In the post-Iraq world, federal spending on federal contracts more than doubled: from $207 billion in 2000 to $500 billion in 2008. The real politics of contracting out is less about contracting than it is about campaign contributions (Witko 2011). According to Scott Amey, general counsel at the project on government oversight, in FY 2008, 60 percent of the contracts were spent on services. While in the past contracts were short term and flexible, "[N]ow they go for 50 years" said Amey (Shane and Nixon 2007).

Contractors work hand-in-glove with the "hybrid" agencies, collect income taxes, and work on agency budgets. They take notes at meetings on war and peace, have a role in intelligence gathering, and fulfill all kinds of security needs in Iraq. Indeed, many functions, from garbage collection to public health and safety to foreign policy, are now being contracted out, creating a vast array of opportunities for those with the wherewithal to take advantage of them. And, few Americans are taking note even when services that

---

[11] See also Ingle, Bob and Sandy McClure, *The Soprano State: New Jersey's Culture of Corruption* (New York: St Martin's Press, 2008).

[12] The estimates were provided by Max Stier, president and CEO of the nonpartisan partnership for Public Services.

have traditionally fallen to the public sector—such as intelligence collection—are contracted out.

Questions about oversight, accountability, and governance inevitably arise. Today, a perfect storm of privatization, globalization, and lack of governmental oversight is taking its toll on community and individual health in America. Government has become so "lean" that it has neither the desire nor the capacity to meaningfully oversee or regulate critical areas of public life. As a result, the list of *Escherichia coli-* and *Salmonella-*contaminated food keeps growing. Tainted produce and food products, from peanuts to cantaloupe to spinach to eggs, routinely find their way to the grocery markets. Similar catastrophes, such as the arthritis drug that caused heart attacks, have plagued the American drug market. At the same time, there are those who argue that the continued growth of uninsured Americans is also a failure of the government, leading to efforts to reform the healthcare system on the national level: first in 1994 under the Clinton administration and again in 2009 during the Obama administration.

Another casualty of the privatization and outsourcing wave was the Walter Reed Hospital scandal. Reporters Dana Priest and Anne Hall of the *Washington Post* revealed the abysmal conditions to which war veterans were subjected at Walter Reed. Their report detailed how 700 veterans endured conditions "nearly as chaotic as the battlefields they faced overseas" along with bureaucratic delays, medical neglect, mouse droppings, and mold (Priest and Hall 2007). At the same time, the progressive privatization of functions was yet another scandal to hit the recently closed hospital. The Army's recommendation was to keep these functions in-house. Later, the Office of Management and Budget protested, and the Army revised its position. A private company, International American Products (IAP), was awarded a $120 million contract that was forged in secrecy. IAP, which was given the charge of the operation and maintenance of Walter Reed, is the same company that provided services in New Orleans after Hurricane Katrina and in Iraq. IAP had patronage ties with the Bush administration through former Treasury Secretary John Snow.

Secrecy and ambiguity also surrounded government contracts, providing the perfect opportunity for political patronage. A $500 million government contract for providing trailer homes to the survivors of Katrina, for example, was awarded on a no-bid basis, similar to many government contracts. These trailer homes were later revealed to have high levels of formaldehyde, a dangerous carcinogen that affected the health of thousands of people. Again, the private contractor was politically well-connected and involved with both the Republican and Democratic political parties.[13]

Hybrids, similar to public agencies, have also become fertile ground for political patronage given the absence of meaningful regulation to affect their governance.[14] The hybrids, or quasi-governmental organizations, are public–private partnerships and are usually defined as those organizations that have some legal relationship or association with the federal government. Also known as "quagos" or "quangos," these organizations include quasi-official agencies (i.e., the Legal Services Corporation, Smithsonian

---

[13] James Varney, "Trailer Dealer May Avoid Fine, Taxes," *Times-Picayune*, September 19, 2006; Eric Lipton, "Governor's Relative is Big Contract Winner," *The New York Times*, December 7, 2006; Sue Sturgis, "Katrina Trailer Contractor Failed to Act on Known Health Risks," *Southern Studies*, July 10, 2006, http://www.southernstudies.org/2008/07/katrina-trailer-contractor-failed-to.html; and Katrina Information, "Key Corporations Cited by House Oversight Committee," http://www.katrinaaction.org/Katrina_contractors.
[14] No one knows for sure, but the hybrids offer a fertile field for new and probing research.

Institution, State Justice Institute, and U.S. Institute for Peace), government-sponsored enterprises (i.e., the Federal National Mortgage Association, known as Fannie Mae, the Federal Home Loan Mortgage Corporation, known as Freddie Mac, and the Federal Agricultural Mortgage Corporation, known as Farmer Mac), federally funded research and development corporations (i.e., Rand, Mitre, and the Institute of Defense Analysis), agency-related nonprofit organizations, venture capital funds, and congressionally chartered nonprofit organizations (Kosar 2011).

Many of the hybrids were created because of the government's concern over protecting the interests of the taxpayers, which could conflict with the interests of private shareholders. This meant government would no longer be competing with businesses, putting the public sector in a better position of helping American businesses to flourish, grow, and pay taxes. But at the same time, the shift toward hybrids also created flourishing opportunities for doling out lucrative contracts to political supporters in lieu of low-level jobs. Moreover, hybrids enjoy privileges not accorded to their competitors in the private sector. Hybrids retain their right to make political contributions, do not need to pay state and local taxes, and are even exempt from paying registration fees to the Securities and Exchange Commission (SEC). In addition, at the behest of the Treasury Department, these agencies can borrow unlimited amounts of money at lower interest rates from the credit markets and the Treasury Department (Kosar 2011, 12). Hybrids are now being created to help expand access to healthcare. Under the Patient Protection and Affordable Care Act, passed in 2009, the Obama administration has sought to fix the chronic challenges facing healthcare in the United States, and has chosen to do so through new policies to expand healthcare to all Americans (Pear 2009).

According to Seidman (1998), most of the "sub-governments" or hybrids conduct their activities largely out of sight of the public, and remain virtually without oversight or scrutiny. Moreover, many of the hybrids, according to Kevin Kosar of the Congressional Research Service, generate their own revenues and do not require government funding. Congressional oversight of the hybrids has been scant. Fannie Mae and Freddie Mac— the two hybrid agencies set up to insure homeowners against mortgage losses that were virtually exempt from either Congressional or public scrutiny—are cases in point.[15] The lobbyists working for Fannie Mae and Freddie Mac successfully lobbied against any supervision or scrutiny that perhaps could have stemmed the financial meltdown in both agencies (Shin 2006). Together, Fannie Mae and Freddie Mac hold more than half of the country's mortgages. In the expectation that the housing market would keep appreciating, these two hybrid agencies encouraged people without adequate assets or stable jobs to buy homes that were clearly beyond their means (Hilzenrath and Goldfarb 2008). The patronage rewards at Fannie Mae and Freddie Mac remained largely out of public view until the economic crisis struck in 2008.

The ambiguities involved in the privatization of war and foreign policy pale in comparison with the political opportunities afforded to organizations fortunate enough to take advantage of the new policies. Companies like Blackwater and Halliburton benefited from their political connections. In the case of Blackwater, the company's founder Erik Prince (together with his family) donated more than $325,000 primarily to the Republican Party. Similarly, Halliburton remained an important defense and health

[15] Today, Fannie Mae and Freddie Mac are viewed as too big and powerful to be effectively regulated and supervised. See Julie Kosterlitz, "Siblings Fat and Sassy: Now That Fannie Mae and Freddie Mac have ballooned into Multibillion-Dollar Players in the Nation's Financial Market, Critics Say These Government Created Companies Are Too Big and Too Powerful," *National Journal* 32 (20) (2000): 1489-1507.

contractor whose livelihood and existence depended on the generosity of the taxpayers. Healthcare contracts—usually smaller than billion-dollar defense contracts—are routinely awarded as no-bid contracts. A 2.8 billion dollar federal no-bid contract on smallpox antiviral medicine suspected to have been awarded through patronage connections, for example, is currently being investigated.[16]

Effects of Patronage in Politics

As is evident, patronage can indeed distort government priorities that often depended on the policy involved. Supporters of NAFTA (The North American Free Trade Act), for example, thought President Clinton's use of patronage to win the vote was a worthy use of presidential prerogatives. But Representative Marcy Kaptur, an Ohio Democrat, was in tears on the House floor during the vote, when she discovered that many colleagues who had pledged to support her opposition to NAFTA had yielded to the White House's blandishments.

Patronage remains an inextricable part of the texture of democratic politics. It is a tool that can be used for good or ill, for progress or repression. In fact, patronage has long been a two-edged sword in politics. It has been used to enact healthcare legislation and prolong wars, prohibit smoking in public places and end term limits, enact programs for the poor, and deprive opponents of jobs. But patronage is also extremely susceptible to corruption—extortion, kickbacks, fraud, and waste, including "no-show" jobs and unnecessary services and projects.

To its critics, political patronage represents the dark underbelly of American politics, whose practitioners are fortunate to keep one step ahead of the sheriff. They believe that patronage breeds corruption, incompetence, and waste. They cite billions in wasted dollars spent on unneeded projects to win political support and the withholding of needed projects to punish political foes. To its practitioners, however, patronage is an essential ingredient of effective government, and those who disdain its use often find themselves unable to enact and implement their programs. They acknowledge the waste, fraud, and abuse inherent in some traditional patronage practices, but say that those practices represent the costs of living in a democracy, where people have freedom of choice. Indeed, as Tip O'Neill noted, patronage is an essential tool of governing. Those who turn up their noses at patronage, like President Carter, often have a difficult time achieving their policy goals. Patronage power is, therefore, defended as a necessary and legitimate extension of the power of elected officials, who must overcome inertia, powerful interest groups, and recalcitrant legislators. A President is not a general, whose orders must be obeyed; on the contrary, his greatest power, according to presidential scholar Richard Neustadt (who had been an aide to President Truman), was the power to persuade.[17]

---

[16] See Brian Bennett, "Victims of an Outsourced War," *Time*, July 19, 2008; Government Accountability Office, "Contingency Contracting—DOD, Kstate, and USAID Contracts and Contractor Personnel in Iraq and Afghanistan," October 2008; Scott Honiberg and Jeffrey Weinstein, "No-Bid Contracts and the Age of Transparency," *Media Health Leaders*, May 10, 2010; Eamon Javers, "House Panels Probing Contract Awarded to Perelman-Affiliated Company," *CNBC*, June 13, 2011.

[17] Richard Neustadt, *Presidential Power: The Politics of Leadership, with Reflections on Johnson and Nixon* (New York: John Wiley & Sons, 1976).

Patronage is a potent tool in that arsenal, with the American people and their elected representatives the obvious targets.

Patronage often encourages public officials to compromise the public interest for private gain and to sacrifice the interests of citizens on the altar of a politician's needs. Why should a neighborhood lose a playground because it voted against a mayor or elected a councilman who refuses to bow to a mayor's wishes? Patronage exists because of human nature and the universal desire for self-improvement. It is both an extension of the electoral process, providing public officials with the tools to govern, and a diminution of the electoral process, robbing legislators of the ability to decide issues solely on their merits. Finally, it is a totally integrated system, in which favors granted by politicians have profound effects upon the selection of national leaders, the goals they achieve, and the future of the nation. With pinstripe patronage, the stakes have soared, with impacts felt around the world.

Conflicts in Health Policy

References

Eggen, Dan, and Paul Kane. 2007. "House GOP Stands Behind Gonzales; New Details of White House Pressure to Fire U.S. Attorneys Do Not Sway Republicans." *Washington Post*, May 11, sec. A-04.

Emanuel, Rahm. 2007. "Don't Get Rid of Earmarks." *The New York Times*, August 24.

Hilzenrath, David S., and Zachary A. Goldfarb. 2008. "Mortgage Giants' Mess Falls to Their Regulator." *Washington Post*, September 11, D-1 and D-3.

Johnson, Carrie. 2008. "Obama Team Faces Major Task in Justice Department Overhaul." *Washington Post*, November 13, sec. A-2.

Kosar, Kevin R. 2011. *The Quasi Government: Hybrid Organizations with both Government and Private Sector Legal Characteristics*. Washington, DC: Congressional Research Service.

Margolin, Josh, and Kelly Heyboer. 2005. "UMDNJ Scandal: With Campus Attorney's Exit, A Star is Done." *The Star-Ledger*, December 23.

Pear, Robert. 2009. "Senate Passes Healthcare Overhaul on Party-Line Vote." *New York Times*, December 24.

Priest, Dana, and Anne Hall. 2007. "Soldiers Face Neglect and Frustration at Army's Top Medical Facility." *Washington Post*, February 18, sec. A-1.

Seidman, Harold. 1998. *Politics, Position and Power*. New York, NY: Oxford University Press.

Shane, Scott, and Ron Nixon. 2007. "In Washington, Contractors Take on Biggest Role Ever." *The New York Times*, February 4, sec. 1-5.

Shin, Annys. 2006. "Examining Fannie Mae—How a Former Chief Helped Shape the Company's Political Culture." *Washington Post*, May 24, sec. D-1.

Tolchin, Martin, and Susan Tolchin. 1972. *To the Victor—Political Patronage from the Clubhouse to the White House*. New York, NY: Random House.

Witko, Christopher. 2011. "Campaign Contributions, Access, and Government Contracting." *Journal of Public Administration Research and Theory* 21 (4): 761-778.

195

www.ingramcontent.com/pod-product-compliance
Lightning Source LLC
Chambersburg PA
CBHW022106280326

41933CB00007B/277